THE REBOOT CLASSROOM

Teacher Decisions in the Time of Covid -19

THE REBOOT CLASSROOM

Teacher Decisions in the Time of Covid-19

Sean Cain • Mike Laird

CONTENTS

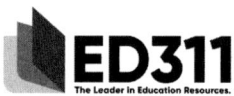

Dedication

This book is dedicated to classroom teachers.
We recognize that despite the rhetoric and because of the mandates,
the weight of successfully rebooting schools
rests squarely on your shoulders.

Thank you for your continued, yet unheralded, service.

AUTHORS' NOTE

This book, *The Reboot Classroom: Teacher Decisions in the Time of Covid-19*, is the companion to the book, *The Reboot: School Operations in an Unpredictable World*. *The Reboot* was written as we were working with school leaders on the problems that need to be addressed and solved regarding the safe reopening of schools during the Covid-19 pandemic. Since the publication of that book, we have received a volume of inquiries from teachers, asking what they can do to protect both themselves and their students when they return to the classroom. That excellent question is the genesis of this book. We put ourselves back in our classroom teacher shoes with our current knowledge of Covid-19, and we have outlined the practices, actions, processes, and procedures we would implement in our personal classrooms when school reopens.

We must clearly state that neither of us is a medical professional or scientist. We are veteran educators and school leaders who understand that at some point schools will reopen and teachers and students will return to the classrooms. As such, from the day schools first closed in March 2020, we have been consumers of the evolving facts and information relating to Covid-19. We have filtered that information through the operational necessity of rebooting schools in a healthy, hygienic, and practical manner.

Clearly, the current Covid-19 crisis is an unprecedented and fluid situation. Ideas and recommendations shared in this book that would be appropriate in one classroom may not be feasible in a different classroom. As we have already experienced, a preventive practice that is identified as reasonable and prudent on one day, is discarded and replaced with a better practice the next day. Much like instructional practice, but at a more rapid pace and with significantly higher stakes. As such, the intent of this book is to not be definitive. The purpose of this book is to serve as a resource for teachers as they prepare to teach effectively in a more safe and hygienic classroom.

Teach forward and wash your hands!
Sean Cain and Mike Laird

Chapter 1

INTRODUCTION

What can one teacher do? A lot!

When schools reopen in the fall, by necessity, things will be different. Many previous daily routines will be abandoned, those daily routines that remain will have new, sometimes significant wrinkles added to them, and a host of entirely new daily routines will need to be adopted. Simple tasks that previously were never consciously considered will take center stage. These tasks include but are not limited to: how students and staff maintain safe distances; how they move and congregate throughout the day; and how classrooms are regularly and effectively sanitized. Without question—fair or not—the work of implementing, monitoring, and managing these new and/or revised processes and practices will fall squarely on the shoulders of teachers.

But honestly, who better to do this? For these new processes and practices to be quickly and effectively implemented requires proactive, purposeful, and on-going explanations, modeling, practice, support, monitoring, and spiraling. Going forward, schools will only become healthier, more hygienic, and more safe through effective instruction delivered to students by their trusted teachers. As teachers, we must embrace the mindset that safely teaching in this time of Covid-19 is not a sprinting exercise. This is a marathon. In the course of this marathon, the health and safety of those in our classrooms will be most impacted by our ability to do the little things right, day in and day out.

There are three guiding principles upon which the recommendations in this book rest. These principles should also guide teacher decision making in the time of Covid-19. The first guiding principle is the understanding that the overarching priorities of a school, and by extension the classroom, have significantly changed. When schools reopen there are only three primary priorities.

Priority A-1: Keep the Adults Alive
Priority A-2: Keep the Students Healthy
Priority A-3: Keep the School Open

The above are the entirety of "A" priorities for the upcoming school year. They are also listed in order of importance. **Keep the Adults Alive** is the recognition that the people most at risk from Covid-19 on a campus are the adults. Yes, students can be infected by Covid-19. However, statistically, they have a better chance of being both asymptomatic and quickly recovering. Adults are more at risk of experiencing more symptoms and serious consequences. The risk of Covid-19 being a person's cause of death increases with age and underlying heath conditions. As a profession, educators are older than the overall population, and many in our profession have underlying health conditions.

Keep the Students Healthy recognizes that students are susceptible to Covid-19. Regardless of the fact that they are less at risk than the adults on campus, they are still at risk. Additionally, even if a student contracts Covid-19 and is fortunate enough to have an asymptomatic case, they can still spread the virus to others, both students and adults. Therefore, by implementing practices and procedures that **Keep the Students Heathy**, the school is also doing the things that are necessary to **Keep the Adults Alive**.

Students need to be in school. In all likelihood, once schools reopen, they will not shutdown wholesale. Instead, individual campuses will close if there is a Covid-19 outbreak on the campus, while other schools remain open. Therefore, schools must implement practices and procedures that guard the overall health and hygiene of those on campus in order to **Keep the School Open**. The by-product of implementing the health and hygiene practices that **Keep the School Open** is that this course of action should also help **Keep the Students Healthy**, representing a viable plan of action to **Keep the Adults Alive**.

The second of the three new guiding principles is the recognition that how schools and classrooms operated prior to March 2020 represents the most unhealthy and unhygienic practices in which we can engage. Not because educators wanted people to get sick, but because previously schools were driven by different goals. Goals that revolved around mass movement, labor efficiency, managing limited budgets, and maximizing academic performance. Schools' goals and priorities have since changed. Going forward, as it relates to health and hygiene practices, pre-March 2020 is now the unacceptable baseline. Build from that low floor, both individually and campuswide. Perfect is not the target. Instead the target is more and better, *more* practices that promote health and hygiene, and practices that *better* promote health and hygiene.

The final guiding principle is risk reduction. The most risk free practice in a pandemic setting is to completely quarantine. Complete quarantine, as we have experienced as a country, is a short-term, imperfect solution. Once we leave our house during a pandemic environment, we assume risks. Once we return to our classroom, we will assume additional risks. As such, we must endeavor to make those activities less risky. We accomplish this by engaging in preventive, healthy, and hygienic practices while away from our homes and in our classrooms.

A useful mental model for risk reduction is to think of a simple dice game. In this dice game only one die is used, and the goal of the game is to NOT roll a 6. Rolling a 6 means that the player loses the game. Rolling any other number is a positive outcome that either allows the player to walk away a winner or to continue playing the game. The optimal strategy for winning the game (not rolling a 6) is to roll the die as few times as possible because every roll of the die represents an additional opportunity to roll a 6 and lose. Figure 1.1 shows the odds of rolling a 6 (losing the game) based on the number of rolls the player attempts.

As figure 1.1 illustrates, if the die is never rolled, the chance of rolling a 6 is 0%. Roll the die only once, and there is a 17% chance of rolling a 6 and losing the game. Continue to roll the die and the odds of losing continue to increase, up to 89% if the die is rolled twelve times. In an environment where we are trying to protect staff and students from a contagion, the goal is to reduce the opportuni-

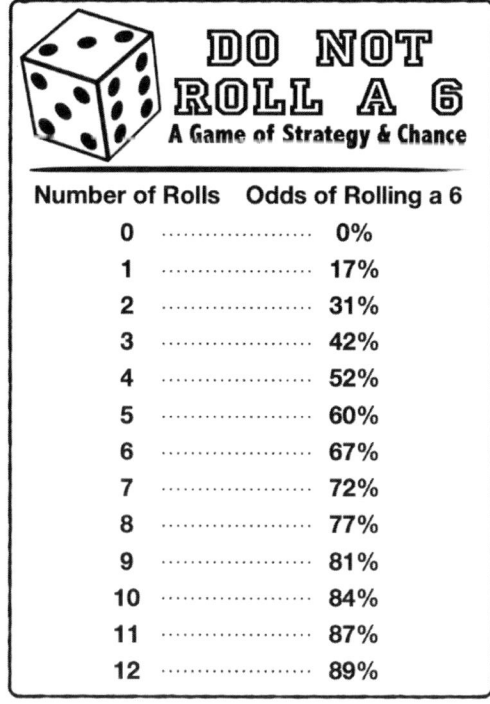

DO NOT ROLL A 6
A Game of Strategy & Chance

Number of Rolls	Odds of Rolling a 6
0	0%
1	17%
2	31%
3	42%
4	52%
5	60%
6	67%
7	72%
8	77%
9	81%
10	84%
11	87%
12	89%

Figure 1.1

ties for risk of infection. Not washing your hands is the equivalent of rolling the die. Not wearing a face mask is rolling the die once again, and so on. Not doing those things (handwashing, face mask wearing, etc.) does not mean that a person will definitely be infected with Covid-19. However, that person is at greater risk for catching Covid-19 than the person who does wash their hands regularly and wears a face mask. Once teachers and students return to the classroom, the safest course of action is to aggressively work to roll the die less often.

Before teachers return to the classroom, they should have a working understanding of how Covid-19 is transmitted; understand how to set up their classroom to improve and enhance health and hygiene; know how to implement quick screening practices to better prevent a person with Covid-19 from having prolonged contact with uninfected students and staff; be able to implement healthy and hygienic classroom practices and procedures for staff and students; and use effective instructional practices for both face-to-face instruction and remote teaching. Reading this book will enhance that understanding.

Chapter 2

PANDEMICS, INCLUDING COVID-19

Pandemics are not new to human history. It has only been in fortunate countries during the past century that the scourge of a pandemic was no longer a part of the life of the typical person. We citizens in developed countries have been the beneficiaries of modern science and medicine. As such, a primer on how pandemics generally play out is a logical place to begin.

Historically, pandemics generally end in one of three ways. A pandemic can end as a result of a medical miracle. Science and medicine develop a successful cure or preventive measure. Two examples of this include smallpox and polio. In both cases, a vaccine was developed that prevented people from contracting the disease, to the point where both diseases have been effectively eradicated. The medical miracle is the best case scenario. But this is also a rare occurrence and can take a long time. As educators, the prudent course of action is to pray for a vaccine but plan as if it will not materialize. This is especially true for the short-run.

The second way a pandemic can end is when the contagion mutates into a less lethal strain. This is not uncommon. As an example, there are still strains of the Spanish Flu that continue to flare up. However, these mutated strains are less deadly to the overall population than the original form of the virus that burned across the globe from 1918 to 1920. Waiting for a contagion to mutate into a less lethal form is time consuming and not guaranteed. Again, for educators, the prudent course of action is to plan as if this will not occur.

The third way that a pandemic can end is through change in human behavior. People realize that the contagion is now part of the daily risk of life and begin to avoid behaviors that increase the risk of contracting the disease and engage in new behaviors that reduce the risk of contracting the disease. Changing behaviors can be difficult and seemingly time consuming. But changing behaviors can be much quicker than waiting on Mother Nature (natural mutation), and it can prevent more cases of the disease and subsequent deaths than waiting patiently for a possible cure (medical miracle).

Ending a pandemic through behavior change could be reason for optimism. Mass behavior change would require a cadre of enthusiastic control freaks who spend their entire career training on how to better get large numbers of people to engage in practices that improve their lives, voluntarily, day after day… If only such people existed and were available.

Now more than ever, the country needs teachers. Teachers are trained to change human behavior, and they do this well with limited resources and next to no fanfare. We believe that closing schools in March was the right thing to do. We also believe that the reason the country is struggling with adopting new behaviors to combat Covid-19 is because the people best suited to drive the necessary changes in daily behavior have been sidelined. This is why schools need to reopen—**safely**—and teachers need to return to the classroom—**safely**. The experts at producing mass behavior change must get back to work at changing behaviors.

Safely reopening schools means that the adults in those schools need to understand how Covid-19 spreads. The most common way the virus is spread is by a person breathing in a large enough dose of the virus to become infected. This is primarily a function of proximity, time, and air volume. The short explanation of this is that the closer the proximity between a non-infected and an infected person, the longer a non-infected person is in contact with an infected person, and the more confined the space where this contact occurs, the greater the chance of a non-infected person becoming infected.

The recommended practices of social distancing, frequent hand washing, face mask wearing, and being outdoors effectively reduce the risk of Covid-19 transmission and infection. Individually, and as a group, these practices reduce the potential of a person being exposed to a large enough virus load to actually become infected. Essentially, when a teacher (or better still, a campus staff) engages in these practices, they are purposefully rolling the die less often. This is why regardless of what the district or campus is doing, we recommend that in the classroom students spread out as much as possible, teachers and students wash their hands frequently, teachers and students wear a face mask, and if there is a window in the classroom that can be opened, it should be open whenever possible.

What can one teacher do? A lot!

Chapter 3

THE CLASSROOM LOFT

C lassroom setup when teachers return to work will represent a significant change from what was customary prior to the March 2020 school closures. As such, we suggest some quick mental preparation before beginning to address this topic. We encourage the reader to take a deep breath. Now, let it out.

It has been our experience that many teachers find the discussion about room setup to be stressful. This is okay. Classroom setup going forward will be a departure from "business as usual." This is a manifestation of the fact that the three most important priorities for this school year are now: **1 - Keep the Adults Alive**; **2 - Keep the Students Heathy**; and **3 - Keep the School Open**. The decisions teachers make this year as they decide how they will set up their classroom will either facilitate the successful fulfillment of these priorities or create environments that put meeting those priorities in jeopardy. Simply put, setting up a classroom with a focus on health and hygiene is a proactive preventive measure and a concrete example of rolling the die less often.

We have observed over the course of our careers that many classrooms begin the year disorganized, cluttered, over-supplied, and under-cleaned. As the school year progresses, this initial situation does not improve. It actually gets worse. Even if a teacher's classroom is not as bad as described, maintaining health and hygiene integrity has never been part of the profession's decision making process. Instead, typical classroom setup decisions were driven primarily by tradition, habit, comfort, convenience, and peer and organizational pressure. This has resulted in cluttered, disorganized classrooms with an excessive amount of instructional and personal materials. This has made the typical classroom essentially impossible to deep clean. This is not the fault of custodial staff; they simply try to clean what is presented.

That was the past. It is time to do better. We have complete confidence that teachers will recognize that due to current circumstances, improved classroom organization and cleanliness is an obligation to protect the health of students and staff. With that recognition, they will put aside their personal and legitimate feelings of discomfort, and they will endeavor to set up their classrooms based on our new shared reality. Additionally, many of the purposeful changes teachers will make to facilitate the health and hygiene of their classroom will also have the added benefit of making their classrooms more conducive to improved student performance. When this is the case, it will be noted.

A useful mental picture for the rebooted classroom is one of a purposefully designed **educational loft**—a space that is sparse of décor and easy to clean while remaining inviting. To implement this picture, teachers will need to re-evaluate their previous room setup opinions and decisions. Those that do not fit within the parameters of what is now required for instructional environments should be discarded. Now all room setup decisions should be viewed and evaluated through the lens of maintaining the **health and hygiene integrity** of the classroom and, by extension, the entire campus. To continue the dice game analogy, the more healthy and hygienically a classroom is initially set up and maintained, the fewer times during the day staff and students are rolling the die, decreasing the chance of rolling a 6.

Teachers should begin with the understanding that from this day forward, **less is more**. The less that is in a classroom, the more that relative space in the classroom is increased. This is critical. We know that increasing the distance between people reduces the chance of a person infected with Covid-19 from spreading the virus to others. Though providing a full six feet of separation between people in a classroom may not be possible, any increase in separation is an improvement over no separation. Previously, it was not uncommon to crowd students in a classroom like so many sardines. This year, any additional spacing that can be created is a step in the right direction. Additionally, by increasing the amount of relative floor space in the classroom, it will be easier for teachers to move around the room efficiently and unobstructed.

The less there is in a classroom, the less there is to clean. This too is critical. When there is less to clean, cleaning can be completed more efficiently, more effectively, and more often. Regular and ongoing effective and efficient cleaning will significantly enhance the health and hygiene of the classroom.

Once the concept of less is more is accepted, natural follow-up questions are *how is this accomplished* and *what does this look like*? To begin, we recommend the campus adopt a standard teacher furnishing package. A single desk, chair, bookcase, file cabinet, and equipment cart will suffice. All other district owned furnishings in the classroom should be removed. Additionally, all teacher owned furnishings should be taken home. This reduction in classroom furnishings will increase relative space in the classroom (in many cases significantly) and increase room cleaning efficiency and effectiveness.

The amount of instructional equipment in the classroom should be reduced. The prevailing practice has been to equip every classroom at the beginning of the school year with all of the instructional equipment that a teacher may need at any time during the year. All of this instructional equipment takes up a lot of space and is rarely, if ever, cleaned during the school year. Now the only instructional equipment that should be in the classroom is the equipment that the teacher uses daily. All other instructional equipment should be gathered, inventoried, and stored in a centralized campus location. Teachers then check out a piece of instructional equipment when they need it and return it when they have finished using it. Additionally, all broken and obsolete instructional equipment should be removed. Far too many observed classrooms take on the appearance of a salvage yard or museum based on the volume of broken equipment and instructional artifacts that are never removed from classrooms. Yes, this includes the combination TV/VCR that was mounted in the corner of the classroom in 1993 and was last used in 1999.

The amount of supplies and materials in a classroom at any given time should be reduced. Much like instructional equipment, many classrooms begin the year stuffed with all the supplies and materials the teacher will need for the entire year. However convenient this may be, this volume of materials takes up space and is rarely, if ever, cleaned. Instead, teachers should keep just enough materials in the classroom that are needed for the week. This does not mean that teachers cannot have all of their supplies and materials; they can. The excess material just cannot be stored in the classroom. This will require teachers to stage their supplies and materials, bringing to class what is needed only as it is needed.

After purposefully removing excess furnishings, equipment, and supplies, the next step is to aggressively remove clutter. Clutter now represents additional things to clean and impediments to efficient room cleaning. Clutter falls into two categories: non-instructional and instructional. Dealing with non-instructional clutter is a relatively straight forward exercise. If an item is non-instructional, remove it from the classroom. The rubric for determining if an instructional item is or is not clutter is driven by the concepts of critical and current. Teachers should ask themselves if a particular item is critical for teaching their content. If the answer is no, then they should remove the item from the classroom. If the answer is yes, then they should ask themselves if the item is critical for the concepts they are currently teaching. If the answer is yes, then the item can remain in the classroom. If the answer is no, then they should remove the item from the classroom. Figure 3.1 is a representation of the teacher decision making process, as it relates to classroom clutter.

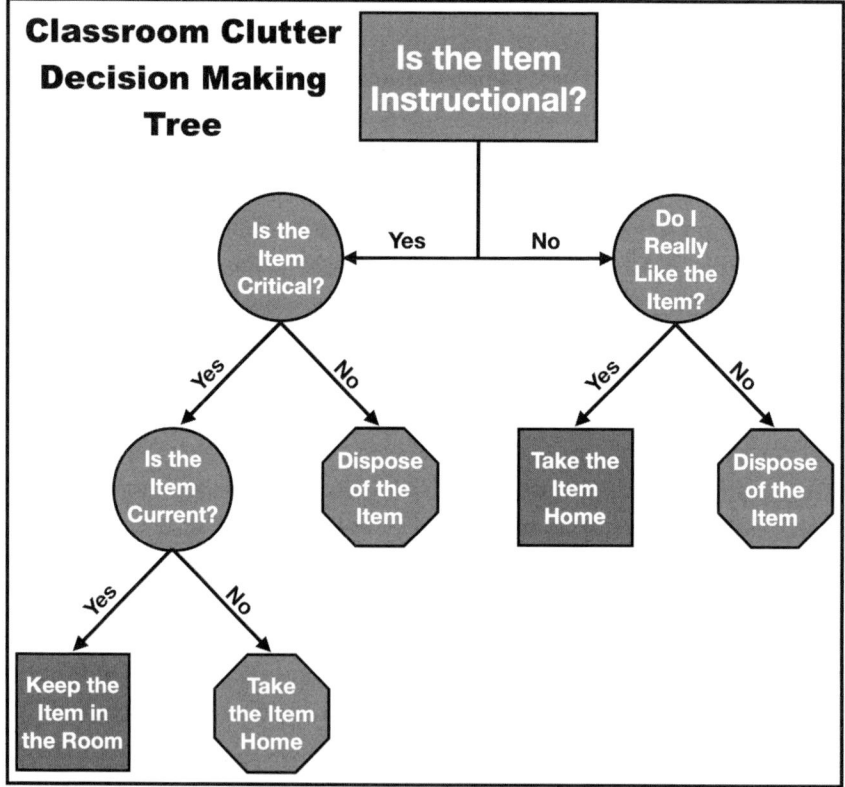

Figure 3.1

Related to the removal of clutter, teachers should also dump their décor. Granted, décor may improve the esthetics and comfort of a classroom, but it is not required for quality instruction. Décor can increase the level of room cleaning difficulty and inefficiency, which in turn can be detrimental to maintaining a healthy and hygienic classroom. No matter how difficult teachers may find this, from not at all to extremely, they can all take comfort in the fact that there is a measurable positive correlation between the lack of clutter and improved student performance. Removing items, cutting clutter, and dumping décor will not hinder instruction. Instead, these actions will enhance it.

Once the removing, cutting, and dumping has been completed, teachers should keep their classrooms (including their workspace) organized. An organized classroom significantly enhances room cleaning effectiveness and efficiency. This is why the loft is the working model of the pandemic era classroom—few items and those few items in their place. For some teachers organization comes easy, and others find this to be more difficult. But regardless of the level of difficulty, increased classroom organization has both hygiene and instructional benefits, including a measurable positive correlation between classroom organization and student performance.

After completing the removing and organizing process, the teacher will be standing in a somewhat sterile classroom. Looking around the classroom, many teachers will be tempted to fill the walls with posters and displays. Resist this temptation. A blank wall is okay. Blank walls can be quickly wiped down and cleaned. When deciding if something is to be placed on the wall, there is a decision making rubric that should be used. First, teachers should ask themselves if the item is instructional. If the answer is no, then do not put the item on the wall. Take the item home instead. If the item is instructional, teachers should ask themselves if the item is critical. Very likely the answer will be no. We have observed that the focus of many instructional wall displays is general and diffused. With such an item the instructional impact is marginal, so there is no need for it to be displayed. If the item is critical to instruction, the final question teachers should ask themselves is if the item is critical to instruction **now**. If yes, the item should be displayed until it is no longer critical. Then that item should be replaced with the next critical and current instructional display.

Figure 3.2 is a representation of the teacher decision making process, as it relates to wall displays. As is the case with furnishings and materials, with wall displays, less is still more. In summary, surfaces that cannot be easily wiped down and sanitized efficiently and effectively represent a potential source of disease transmission. As such, any items that remain in a classroom must be both essential for today's instruction and easy to clean.

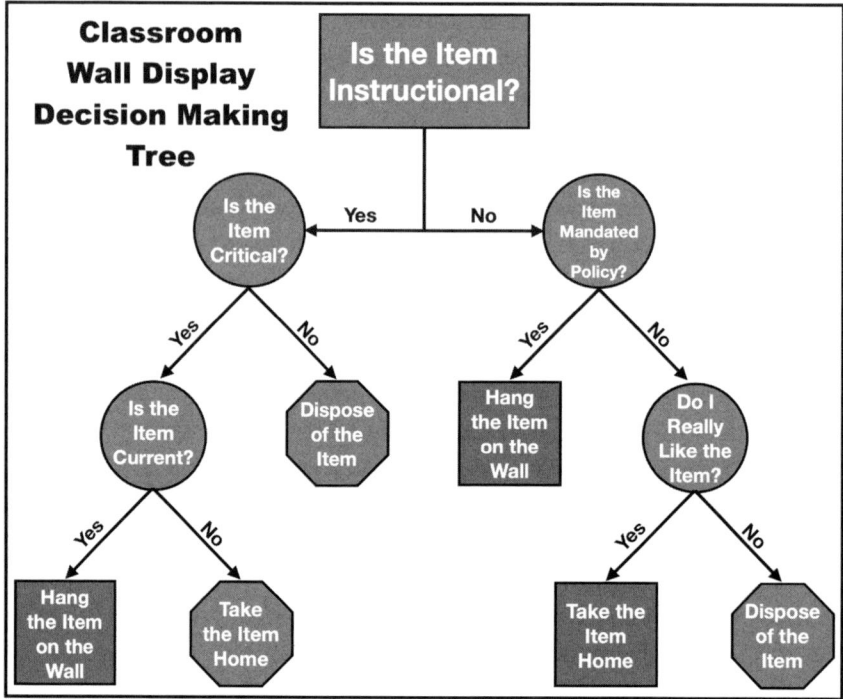

Figure 3.2

The final consideration in classroom setup is windows. For the reader who does not have an exterior window in their classroom, it is okay to skip to the next chapter. For teachers fortunate enough to have an exterior window, here are some things to consider. First, window treatments and blinds should be inspected and evaluated. Window treatments and blinds that are in good condition and can be cleaned quickly and easily can remain. If this is not the case, the offending blinds or window treatments represent a detriment to classroom health and hygiene and should be removed prior to students returning to class.

Once students return to school, window treatments and blinds should remain open as much as possible. The reason for this is because natural light serves as a natural sanitizer. Over time, natural light degrades the virus to the point where it is no longer transmittable. If the window itself can be opened, so much the better, and it should be opened whenever possible. There are three reasons why this is the case. First, filtered natural light (light passing through window glass) is a sanitizer. Unfiltered natural light is an even more effective sanitizer and will degrade the virus at a quicker pace. Second, with an open window there is a steady volume of fresh air entering the room. Increased amounts of fresh air effectively decrease the volume of the Covid-19 virus particles potentially in the classroom, reducing the chance of virus transmission. Finally, with fresh air entering the room through the open window, air circulation within the classroom is improved, potentially reducing the chance of a person breathing in a large enough virus dose to become infected. Needless to say, having an exterior classroom window and utilizing it effectively can significantly enhance the overall health and hygiene of a classroom. There is also an additional instructional benefit. Increased levels of light, especially natural light, have a measurable positive correlation with improved performance.

In summary, when teachers prepare their classrooms for face-to-face instruction this year, they should purposefully reduce the volume of furnishings, equipment, materials, and wall displays in the room. Teachers should refrain from bringing any décor into the room. Teachers should organize what remains in the room and endeavor to keep the room organized throughout the entire school year. If teachers have an exterior widow, they should keep the blinds open as much as possible. If the widow can be opened, it should remain open when possible while students are in the classroom. A room set up in the manner described (see figure 3.3) represents the first step in creating and maintaining a healthy and hygienic instructional environment.

What can one teacher do? A lot!

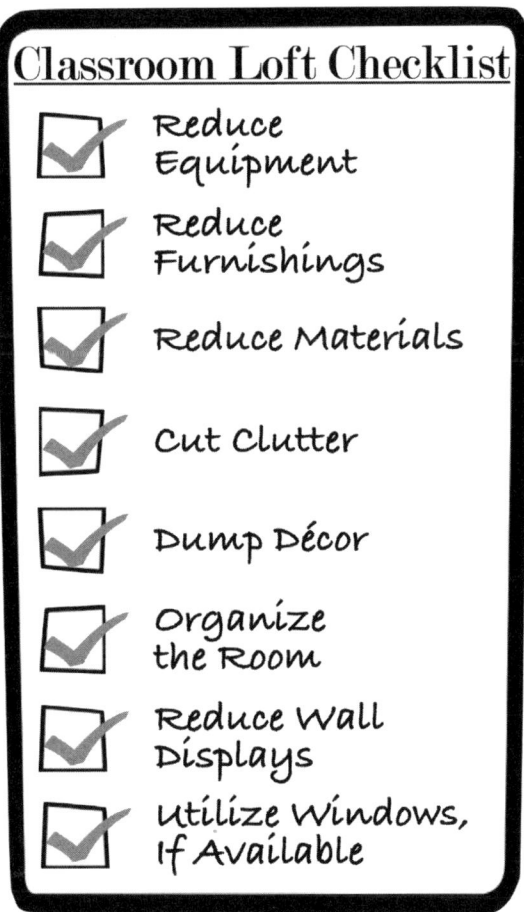

Classroom Loft Checklist

- ☑ Reduce Equipment
- ☑ Reduce Furnishings
- ☑ Reduce Materials
- ☑ Cut Clutter
- ☑ Dump Décor
- ☑ Organize the Room
- ☑ Reduce Wall Displays
- ☑ Utilize Windows, If Available

Figure 3.3

Chapter 4

QUICK HEALTH SCANS

Regardless of campus practice, we recommend that teachers conduct quick, non-intrusive Covid-19 symptom scans in their classrooms throughout the day. We do not make this recommendation in an attempt to circumvent any district and/or campus policy. On the contrary, this recommendation is in recognition that proactive teacher practice will augment the effectiveness of any district and/or campus policy. In a Covid-19 environment, the reality of the situation is that the health and hygiene integrity of the overall campus is actually the sum of individual teacher practice. Also, when teachers conduct regular, non-intrusive Covid-19 symptom scans throughout the day, those teachers will have a higher degree of confidence that they and their students are safe and healthy, thus allowing all of them to better focus on teaching and learning. This final point (an increased level of confidence in shared health and safety) is not made lightly. As schools reopen and staff and students return, until the basic human needs of safety and security—and the psychological needs of connection and relationship—are addressed and fulfilled, teaching and learning will be negatively impacted.[1]

The first and easiest scan a teacher should implement requires an awareness of common Covid-19 symptoms and asking students if they have recently or are currently experiencing any of those symptoms (see figure 4.1). Additionally, teachers should be aware that based on a recent study conducted by the University of Leeds (2020), a persistent cough and fever is the most common presenting symptom combination for those infected with Covid-19. As such, a student developing a cough during class should warrant additional screening.

Second, we recommend that every teacher have an infrared thermometer in their classroom. We are on the record recommending that school

---

[1] Maslow's Hierarchy of Needs (1943): Physiological, Safety, Belongingness and Love, Esteem, Self-actualization.

districts provide these thermometers to all of their teachers. However, we also realize that this recommendation will not be followed by every district and school. For the teacher who works on a campus that does not provide them with an infrared thermometer, they should purchase their own before students return to class. Having to purchase their own thermometer may not be "fair" to teachers, but it is prudent.

The reason why every teacher needs to have an infrared thermometer is so they are able to quickly check the temperature of their students multiple times a day. If the school is not conducting fever scans before students enter the building, then teachers should do their own fever scans when students enter their room. In addition to the first fever scan of the morning,

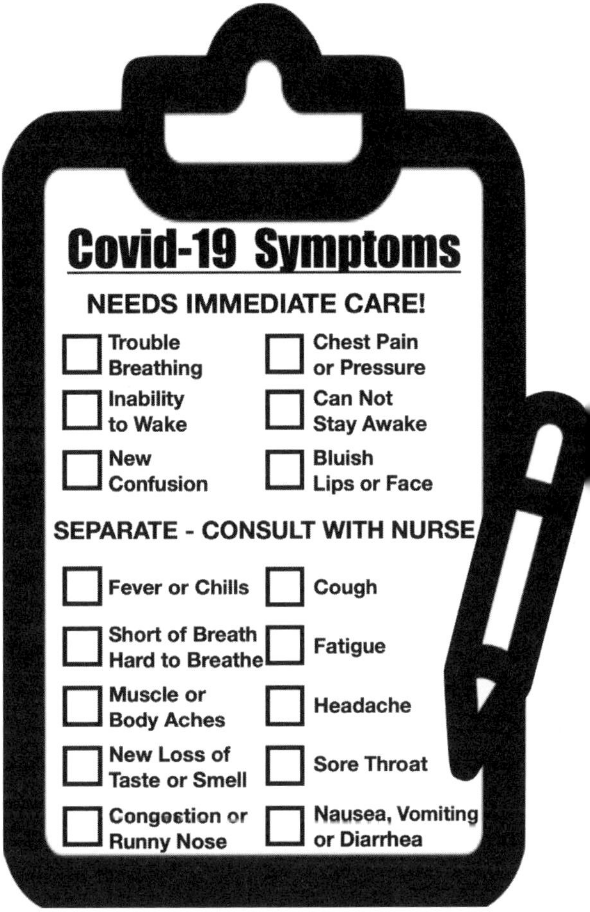

Covid-19 Symptoms

NEEDS IMMEDIATE CARE!

☐ Trouble Breathing   ☐ Chest Pain or Pressure
☐ Inability to Wake   ☐ Can Not Stay Awake
☐ New Confusion   ☐ Bluish Lips or Face

SEPARATE - CONSULT WITH NURSE

☐ Fever or Chills   ☐ Cough
☐ Short of Breath Hard to Breathe   ☐ Fatigue
☐ Muscle or Body Aches   ☐ Headache
☐ New Loss of Taste or Smell   ☐ Sore Throat
☐ Congestion or Runny Nose   ☐ Nausea, Vomiting or Diarrhea

Figure 4.1

teachers at the secondary level should conduct a fever scan every period at the beginning of class. At the elementary level, teachers should conduct fever scans at the beginning of every instructional block and when students return to class from art, music, PE, and other enrichment courses. This is a lot of fever scans and a lot of redundancy. This is by design. Many people infected with Covid-19 initially present as asymptomatic. This seems to be especially true with children. This means that a person can be infected with Covid-19 for an indeterminant amount of time before a symptom appears. Additionally, the first Covid-19 symptom can present at any time during the day or night. Just because a person does not have a fever at the beginning of first period does not mean that they will remain fever free throughout the day. By conducting multiple fever scans, a previously asymptomatic person can be identified in a more timely fashion. This is of critical importance because research indicates that **a person with Covid-19 is most contagious when symptoms first begin to appear**. Identifying someone with Covid-19 earlier makes everyone on campus safer and makes contact tracing less complicated.

Third, teachers should introduce multiple smell scans throughout the day. This is due to the fact that the loss of smell (anosmia) is often an early symptom experienced by a person with Covid-19. Additionally, experiencing anosmia is a more accurate screener (fewer false positives) for Covid-19 than having a fever. A quick smell scan can be potentially less stressful than a fever scan. Students can be asked to smell a scented card, some flowers or plants, or scented hand sanitizer. Those who can do so can enter the class. Those who are unable to smell the aroma of the selected item are separated for additional screening.

It must be understood that screening is not meant to be definitive. Instead, screening is a scalable but imprecise, preventive practice. Being screened and not having a fever, anosmia, and/or presenting with any other symptom does not mean that the person does not have Covid-19. It simply means they are less likely to have the virus than someone with a symptom. Conversely, just because a screened person is found to have a fever, anosmia, and/or any other symptom does not mean they have Covid-19. It simply means that additional information and/or investigation is required to determine if the result of the scan is a false positive or false negative (either being possible) or if further action should be taken.

In short, simply feeling good is not proof that a person is virus free, and feeling bad does not mean that a person has Covid-19. Additionally, an infected person can go from asymptomatic (feeling good) to symptomatic (feeling bad) at any time. This is why multiple scans and multiple types of scans conducted throughout the day add a significant layer of protection and peace of mind for everyone on campus. Redundancy and diligence represent proactive defenses against Covid-19—purposefully rolling the die less.

Chapter 5

CLASSROOM HEALTH AND HYGIENE PRACTICES

O nce the classroom loft is set up and daily screening practices are established and operational, many teachers might ask, "Now can I just focus on instruction?"

The answer is, "Not yet."

Let us refer once again to our guiding priorities for this school year: **1 - Keep the Adults Alive; 2 - Keep the Students Healthy**; and **3 - Keep the School Open**. In meeting these priorities, room setup represents Step 1. Regular screening represents Step 2. The next step is to adopt and implement daily classroom health and hygiene practices by both teachers and students. This chapter will present a slate of rational, manageable, and proactive practices that will maintain and enhance the overall integrity of classroom health and hygiene.

For teachers following the recommendations of this book, they have already completed the first step in building and maintaining a healthy and hygienic classroom. That first step is setting up their classroom "loft" style and then maintaining the classroom loft throughout the year. Practicing the principle of "less is more," eliminating clutter, and keeping the room organized makes the room easy to clean often, quickly, and deeply. Creating more open space allows increased separation between students, lessening both the chance and potential impact of Covid-19 transmission. Utilizing available exterior windows in the classroom allows for the natural sanitizing power of the sun, and opening windows increases the volume of fresh air in the room and improves air circulation. Yet again, reducing the chance of Covid-19 infection. Once these actions are complete, then the classroom is ready for screened students to arrive.

Once students are in the room, maintaining a healthy and hygienic learning environment becomes the single most important priority of the teacher and class. This is what will increase the odds that the school is able to: **1 – Keep the Adults Alive; 2 – Keep the Students Healthy**; and **3 – Keep**

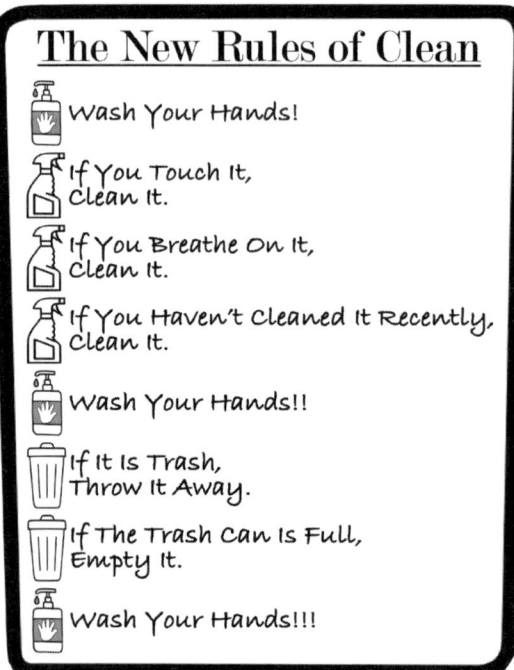

The New Rules of Clean

Wash Your Hands!

If You Touch It,
Clean It.

If You Breathe On It,
Clean It.

If You Haven't Cleaned It Recently,
Clean It.

Wash Your Hands!!

If It Is Trash,
Throw It Away.

If The Trash Can Is Full,
Empty It.

Wash Your Hands!!!

Figure 5.1

the School Open. To achieve this will require a host of cleaning and sanitizing practices by teachers and students that should be adopted in every classroom. A broad summary of those practices are illustrated in figure 5.1.

Before these practices are better explained, we again remind the reader that we do not make these recommendations in an attempt to circumvent any district and/or campus policy. The implementation of these recommendations will augment the effectiveness of any district and/or campus policy. In the rare case where no policy or direction has been provided, the individual teacher is still in a position to create a healthy and hygienic bubble in their classroom. Essentially, in the area of school where a teacher spends most of the workday (their classroom), by implementing regular and consistent classroom health and hygiene procedures, they are purposefully rolling the die less.

1 (Start of Class): At the beginning of each class (instructional block in an elementary setting, class period in a secondary setting), when students arrive they immediately wash their hands.[2] This can be accomplished by either installing hand sanitizer dispensers outside of every classroom or by having hand sanitizer available in the classroom. There are classrooms that have working sinks in them (science labs and many elementary classrooms). In these rooms soap and water hand washing is an option but may prove to be too time consuming. If this is the case, the use of hand sanitizer would be appropriate.

---

[2] Wash hands: Hand washing can either be through the use of soap and water or through the use of a hand sanitizer that is at least 60% alcohol. Of the two options, the use of soap and water is more effective. However, the use of hand sanitizer is generally more convenient, can be used in more settings, and is less time consuming.

2 (Start of Class): Once students have washed their hands, they get a cleaning wipe and wipe down their desk/work area, chair, and materials they will use during class. Once these items have been cleaned, they dispose of the used cleaning wipe in a designated trash can or trash bag.

3 (Start of Class): After disposing of the used cleaning wipe, students once again wash their hands. Now they are ready for class.

Once class begins, any time a student enters the classroom they should again wash their hands. There should be no exceptions to this rule, regardless of where the student has come from, what they were doing, or how long they were gone. It is impossible to determine what the student touched when they were outside the classroom. Therefore, err on the side of caution and prevention and have the student wash their hands… again.

4 (End of Class): At the end of class, the start of class procedures are essentially followed. All students organize and set aside their work and wash their hands.

5 (End of Class): After washing their hands, students get a cleaning wipe and wipe down the materials they used, their desk/work area, and their chair. Once students have cleaned what they used and touched, they dispose of the used cleaning wipe in a designated trash can or trash bag. In lieu of students wiping down the materials they used, there is a second option. The class can have a "used material box." With a "used material box," students place their used materials in the class specific box. The box is then left undisturbed for at least 72 hours (time is a disinfectant). After 72 hours (three days) have elapsed, the items can then be removed from the box, wiped down with a sanitizing wipe, and placed back in service for students to use. If a teacher decides to utilize this option, we recommend using five boxes, one box for each day of the work week. The use of five boxes (labeled for each day of the work week) increases the sanitizing effect of time and prevents confusion about when the materials in a box were last used.

6 (End of Class): After disposing of the used cleaning wipe, students once again wash their hands. Now they are ready to leave the classroom for their next class, where these steps should be repeated.

For the reader who may now think that implementing these procedures will be either too time consuming or that students will be either unable or unwilling to participate, set aside your skepticism. The authors observed the above described routines being used on multiple campuses in K-12 classrooms during February and March 2020, just prior to the nationwide school closures. The process was often completed before the tardy bell rang in secondary classrooms and took less than three minutes at the end of class. In observed elementary classrooms, it was a very important student job to be the person who squirted the hand sanitizer on the hands of classmates, handed out the sanitizing wipes, or went around the room with the trash bag for the used cleaning wipes.

Again, these quick hand cleaning and room sanitization procedures should occur at the beginning and end of every instructional block or segment in elementary schools and at the beginning and end of every period in secondary schools. More simply put, this should occur every 30 to 90 minutes, based on the natural operational rhythms of the school and classroom.

At the end of the school day, or the last period students are in the classroom, teachers should allocate an additional two to five minutes for a final round of room sanitation. In addition to the end of class health and hygiene procedures, students should assist in putting up all equipment and making sure that the room is organized and flat surfaces are empty. Students should also wipe down bookcases, shelves, and other high touch/use areas. Students should pick up and properly dispose of any trash in the room. When this is complete, students wash their hands one last time, and the teacher quickly checks student temperatures and/or checks for anosmia. The room is now clean, students are ready to go home, and another healthy day of school is complete. After students are dismissed, the teacher checks the inventory of cleaning and sanitation supplies, making a note to replace and replenish what is needed, and confirms that the room is ready for deeper cleaning by custodial staff.

Yes, there is considerable redundancy in the procedures described above. That is by design. Redundancy provides an additional layer of protection for both the teacher and students. First, if any step is not completed satisfactorily one time, a distinct possibility, the next time or the next-next time will correct this. Second, if a person infected with Covid-19 is in the classroom, that person is constantly shedding the virus. This is the case even if the person is asymptomatic. By implementing regular and on-going classroom hygiene and cleaning practices, any live virus particles that are shed are more likely to be removed or more quickly degraded, rendering those virus particles no longer contagious.

Yes, these cleaning and sanitizing practices will take time from every instructional block or class period. This will be a constant infringement on instructional time. These practices are also the greatest defenders of instructional time. As the teacher and the class begin to feel confident that the cleaning and sanitation practices they are engaged in are actually protecting their health and well-being while instruction is being delivered, there is a greater chance that learning is taking place. Also, the implementation of these cleaning and sanitation practices will significantly increase the chance that the school will remain open longer which in turn will increase the amount of face-to-face instruction that is delivered. Face-to-face instruction is more effective than remote instruction and infinitely more effective than no instruction. Additionally, the more these cleaning and sanitizing practices become routine, the faster students will complete them. In total, approximately five minutes per class period should be allocated for cleaning and sanitizing practices.

It is also important to note the benefits that classrooms that implement regular cleaning and sanitizing practices create for custodial staff. First, the classrooms that do this have created a safer work environment for the custodial staff. Second, because custodial staff are able to work in a safer environment, their level of stress is potentially reduced. Finally, when custodians are in a room that is orderly, easy to clean, and already surface level cleaned, they are able to clean that room deeper, more effectively, and more efficiently. This in turn makes the classroom healthier, more hygienic, and safer when the teacher and class return to the classroom.

Before moving from the discussion of classroom health and hygiene practices, we must state that it is our sincere hope that schools provide teachers with the supplies they need to adequately enact these practices in every classroom. We also know that this will not always be the case. If a teacher works at a campus that is unable (most likely) or unwilling (less likely) to provide them with cleaning and hygiene supplies, that teacher would be well advised to provide them themself. This will represent an additional (unfair) expense for some teachers, but the additional health, security, and subsequent peace of mind provided by these expenditures will be worth the cost.

The initial robust discussion about the value of face masks that occurred through the spring and early summer has been factually settled. Mandated or not, wearing a face mask is a proactive, preventive measure that reduces the spread of Covid-19. Wearing a face mask provides significant protection to others if the individual wearing the mask has Covid-19, even if the person is asymptomatic. Wearing a face mask provides a level of protection for the mask wearer if they come in contact with an infected person. Wearing a face mask is now a recognized health and hygiene best practice, and when a person does so it becomes yet another example of rolling the die less. Therefore, when students are in the building—in the classroom or not—all teachers, staff, and students should wear a face mask and do so correctly.

In addition to face masks, face shields can also be worn in the classroom. In the course of on-going conversations with school leaders across the country, many of them have indicated that teachers will be provided with and required to use face shields when delivering face-to-face instruction. Many teachers have indicated that they plan on wearing face shields, even if they have to provide their own. If face shields are worn in conjunction with face masks, we support this decision. A face shield provides an additional layer of protection for the wearer, especially if that person is in close contact with an infected person. The face shield can prevent virus laden spray and respiratory droplets from entering the wearer's eyes, a possible source of Covid-19 transmission. However, on its own a face shield provides limited protection from virus particles that the wearer may inhale. The virus particles are simply breathed in with the air that flows around the face shield. With face shield use the equation is simple. **Face shield + face mask = enhanced protection**. Face shield – face mask = limited protection. The final point to make about face masks and face shields is if students are required to wear one or both, the teacher must model the behavior. We are teaching new practices, habits, and routines to students. The daily example set by teachers will be the strongest factor in how quickly and successfully students learn these new practices.

There has been some interest and discussion about teachers wearing medical scrubs as work attire. Though not a strictly preventive practice, this may be something that teachers want to consider. Scrubs are standard dress throughout the health profession. When school resumes, teachers will be more involved in proactively maintaining the health and hygiene integrity of their classrooms. Copying the common practice of health professionals should, at least at face value, be a good idea. Scrubs are fairly inexpensive, durable, provide a level of comfort, and accommodate a wide range of motion. They are also available in a variety of colors and print patterns that could be easily used to reflect school spirit and support esprit de corps. The real value of scrubs is that they are easy to change in and out of quickly, and they are easy to clean and sterilize in the hot water cycle of a washing machine. Teachers who elect to wear scrubs could keep an extra set in their room in case they are involved in an incident where changing clothes would be a prudent course of action.

When conferring with medical professionals in the course of writing this book, it was pointed out that wearing scrubs allowed them (medical professionals) to reduce the chance of transferring contamination from their work into their home. This is accomplished by removing their shoes and soiled scrubs in the garage or laundry room as soon as they get home. This is followed by immediately washing their scrubs, taking a quick shower, and putting on clean clothes. The purpose of this is to reduce by as much as possible the chance of any contagion accidently being brought into the home. If a teacher is serious about wearing scrubs in the classroom for hygiene purposes, they would be well advised to also adopt the described after work practices of medical professionals.

Over the course of rebooting classrooms, there will be more unknowns than knowns. Maintaining the health and hygiene integrity of the classroom is one way to reduce the number of unknowns that will be faced. Well-crafted health, cleaning, and sanitizing procedures executed with a high degree of fidelity will enhance health and safety for everyone in the classroom. This year and for the immediate future, hygiene is the prerequisite for instruction.

What can one teacher do? A lot!

Chapter 6

BUILD A CLASS COMMUNITY

When students return to the classroom, teachers should be ready to address the social and emotional needs of students in a purposeful and proactive manner. Initially, this will take precedence over instruction and will remain an area that requires on-going attention throughout the year. For the reader now thinking, "I am a teacher, not a counselor," that was last year. This year you are both, and for a while, especially at first, academic instruction is several spots down on the priority list. For teachers who love and value the academic component of instruction above all else, this realization may be difficult. Decisions on why and how valuable time from content will be taken to support student emotional health must be openly discussed by staff, and the importance of doing so must be emphasized and reinforced. The truth of the matter is that teachers are the ones that set the tenor and tone of student/adult interactions. Often this occurs in a somewhat fluid and organic manner. Now this needs to be systematic and overt.

Consider what students have experienced and witnessed since March 2020. Schools closed without warning. A pandemic has engulfed the nation and has been a centerpiece of media attention. An unarmed African American man, George Floyd, was killed by a police officer, and it was caught on video. This has been a centerpiece of media attention. Large and sometimes multi-day protests against systemic racism have occurred in cities and towns across the country. This has been a centerpiece of media attention. Family life has been turned upside down due to the school closures, quarantine lockdowns, lost jobs, and the subsequent downturn in the economy. To this, add the students who have dealt with a relative or friend who either survived a serious case of Covid-19, or worse, did not.

This is why, in order of importance, the focus of teachers in classrooms this year is as follows: 1 – Health and Hygiene; 2 – Emotional Health and Belonging; 3 – Academic Instruction. Only after students begin to feel

more safe, become less traumatized, feel less stressed, and begin to re-
connect with fellow students and teachers will learning begin to occur.
Many schools plan to adopt formalized SEL (social emotional learning)
programs and provide teachers with curriculum and lessons that address
student emotional well-being. We encourage this. Other schools will allocate time during the day to specifically address student social-emotional
needs. This too, we encourage. Some schools will decide to do nothing.
Regardless of campus decisions, this year you the teacher are more critical
than any (or lack of any) program. As such, we recommend that classroom
teachers work to implement the following.

Students look to their teachers for guidance. When students know that
their teacher has a plan, can explain the plan, and can justify the plan, their
anxiety is eased. When this plan is evident and demonstrated through daily
routines, the positive effect is magnified. Predictable classroom routines
provide a sense of comfort and consistency for students, and the quicker
a teacher can create a calm and purposeful "normal" in their classroom,
the better. Once established, solid and predictable routines allow everyone
to know what is happening and have a sense of control during the day.
Work to build a sense of team or family in your classroom. Let each student know and feel that they are part of something bigger than themselves.
Do this purposefully. Greet your students as they enter the room. Where
previously a pat on the back and smile would suffice, now this requires a
quick fever scan and warm words. Do this every day. Celebrate the lack
of a fever, point out that the student is back for another healthy day, and
be enthusiastic about having them in the class. These actions are concrete
examples that demonstrate to students how much the teacher cares about
them.

On the first day of class, do not worry about instruction. Instead, let
each student introduce themselves. Honestly address that things are now
different and that it is okay to be anxious. Share with students why the
classroom is set up the way that it is and the benefit of the new setup.
Talk about the scanning routines that are in place in your classroom and
why this is important to keep everyone safe and healthy. Explain, model,
and practice the hygiene and sanitation procedures that the entire class
will participate in every day and why it is important that they are active in
keeping themselves, their friends, and their family healthy and safe. Create
a shared classroom social contract that is less focused on *do nots* and more
focused on how people will treat each other, support each other, accept

each other, and talk to each other. Explain that this year your classroom is a judgement free safe space where they will also learn about your content.

Then "walk the talk." Begin each class period with a quick "Class Check-in." During this class check-in time, talk about what students want to talk about. Process with them, guide them, but most of all listen to them. Model how you want students to treat each other and talk to each other. Be inclusive, and do not allow a student in your class to be ostracized. The more you engage positively with every student and the more you overtly treat every student with dignity and respect, the more your students will follow your lead. If after the first few weeks of school a daily Class Check-in is no longer necessary, the frequency can be reduced. However, for this school year, at least one Class Check-in per week is the minimum recommendation.

Teachers should attempt to create a stress free learning environment. Although a little stress can be a good thing, too much stress is toxic. Too much stress has a negative impact on learning, health, mood, and behavior. This year, begin with the assumption that everyone in the classroom is significantly overstressed, including you. Teachers welcoming their students everyday as they enter the classroom is the beginning of a continuous stress reduction process. Having healthy routines that students follow continues this process. Granted, the calming accoutrements and décor that were common in classrooms last year will have been removed. However, many students find clean, organized, and clutter free classrooms to be less claustrophobic and distracting, hence less stressful. Additionally, the teacher can have soft music playing in the background and an open window flooding the room with light and possibly fresh air. These actions often have a positive effect on mood and attitude.

Along with these foundational stress reducing practices, we recommend that teachers adopt additional stress reducing procedures. Once students are settled in their desks, take time to explain what will occur in the class today, even to the point of how much time will be devoted to each activity. Explain to students how they will demonstrate their progress or success by the end of class. Also, ease back on the importance of a grade, especially for the first six to nine weeks of school. What is important is that students acclimate to an eerily similar yet completely different school environment. They need to de-stress, and they need time for the intellectual fog of five or more months of academic regression to lift.

This does not mean that the teacher should water down the academic work that students will engage in while in class. On the contrary, challenging work in itself can provide a distraction and welcome release from other pressures. What we encourage is that the "grades" recorded in the early months of this upcoming school year be more reflective of participation, effort, and progress. The goal of grading this year is not to separate those who have an affinity for a subject from those who do not. The goal of grading this year is to ease students back into an academic mode through a process that recognizes growth and reinforces effort. We go as far as suggesting that for the first six to nine weeks of school, if a student engages in the assigned academic work (from daily work to a test) and gives an honest effort, the lowest numerical score they should receive is a 70. This should be communicated to students in the following way, **"For the first six weeks of this school year, if you try, if you refuse to give up, and if you turn in your work, you will not fail. I promise."**

Understandably, many teachers are concerned about student behavior when school resumes. It is our belief that for the most part, student behavior will be better than expected, with exceptions to this being more noticeable and intense. Most students want to return to school. This return will be like a warm blanket to them, providing a level of comfort, security, and consistency that has been absent in their lives since schools closed in March 2020. There will also be students that are unable to initially process the stress, anger, grief, fear, change, and/or uncertainty that is present in all of our lives at this moment, and they will aggressively act out for seemingly little things, magnifying the inappropriateness of their behavior.

If you doubt this, watch the available videos of how some adults have responded when asked to wear a face mask. The not wearing a face mask is the behavior, the request to wear a face mask is the spark, and the stress, fear, and uncertainty that has been building up in the person is the fuel for their over the top, inappropriate outburst. Afterwards some of these people admit to not recognizing themselves in the video and are extremely embarrassed and apologetic. This is not an excuse for all outlandish adult behavior, just some of it. There are some people who are legitimate jerks.

The point is that teachers cannot be surprised when the misbehavior of a child or teen is actually the manifestation of really big, unaddressed feelings. Instead, teachers should anticipate this and have a plan to first prevent it and then respond to it in an appropriate, nurturing manner. Up to this point, everything discussed in this chapter has been ways that support student emotional health and facilitate a classroom environment that provides a foundation for widespread appropriate student behaviors.

Continuing in this direction, it will be critical for teachers to let go of the all too common adult practice of "Do as I say, not as I do." The most powerful way to teach anything is to model what is being taught. Therefore, for every classroom expectation this year, teachers should adopt the philosophy and practice of "**Do as I do.**" The behaviors, examples, and actions by teachers communicate much more powerfully than their words. If students are expected to wear face masks, then the teacher wears a face mask. If students are expected to clean their desk and materials, then the teacher cleans their desk and materials. If students are expected to speak politely and respectfully, then the teacher speaks politely and respectfully, and so on, with every rule and expectation. For expectations that are new to students, practice them as a group. For example, practice the correct way to wash one's hands, wear a face mask, and clean a desk. Practice walking down the hall with appropriate distancing. The behaviors students pick up quickly require less practice. Some behaviors require more practice and regular refreshers. Keep in mind that behavior practice is not a punishment. Just as math facts practice, spelling words practice, and band practice are not punishments. Practice is simply what we do to improve, regardless of the subject. The more a teacher models expectations and provides opportunities for students to practice expectations, the better overall student behavior becomes.

We suggest that teachers let go of the traditional way of developing classroom rules. This means rules that the teacher developed and presents to the class, mostly written as negatives or behaviors to avoid. *No gum chewing in class* and *no talking without permission* are examples of this. Instead, time during the first day of class should be devoted to developing a classroom social contract. A classroom social contract is a shared agreement between and among the students and teacher addressing how they will treat each other and what behavioral norms they will follow. This shared agreement increases the level of buy-in from students because they had input in its development. In contrast, traditional class rules can be viewed as a set of constraints handed down from on high, which often creates a level of resentment in those being constrained. This is why students are integral in the development of a classroom social contract. Granted, the teacher represents the first among equals in the development of the classroom social contract, and depending on the age and ideas of the students in the class, the teacher may remain the primary force shaping the final product. However, regardless of the level of teacher guidance and shaping, students will see their ideas in the document, and as a result they will feel an increased sense of responsibility to follow it. Figure 6.1 is an example of a class developed social contract.

A good classroom social contract provides a focus on **what to do**, as opposed to **what not to do**. When students know what to do

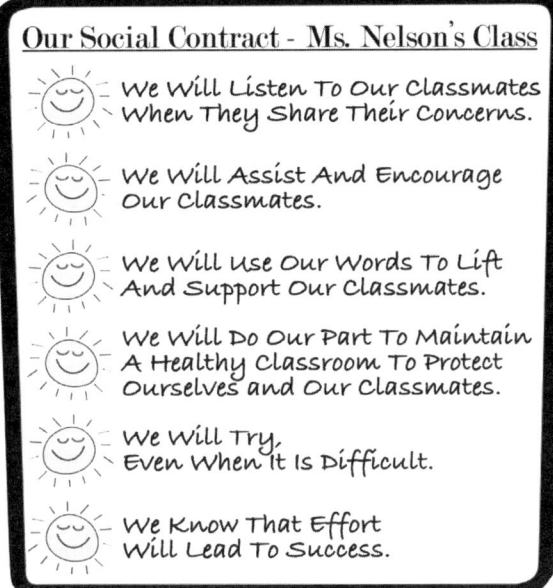

Figure 6.1

and then do those things, it creates a sense of personal empowerment and control. Once the classroom social contract has been developed, post it prominently on the wall. Yes, the classroom social contract is so important that even in a loft style classroom setup it should be displayed. Then the teacher and the class follow the social contract. When necessary, the teacher and the class refer back to it, and if someone strays, the social contract becomes a tool that helps that person right themself.

Doing all that is described above will not extinguish all student misbehavior. Students are human and children. Misbehavior is a given, a part of both the human and child condition. The culture and climate of the classroom and how the teacher responds to the misbehavior are the critical variables. Culture is the body of practices in the classroom and how those practices are enacted. Climate is the positive or negative effect those practices have on students. In spite of what many educators are led to believe, a positive classroom culture and climate does not occur by accident. It is created, managed, and maintained by the teacher.[3] In "normal times"

---

[3] A modified version of Dr. James Davis' definition of campus culture and climate. *Culture is the practices of a campus and the way adults enact those practices. Climate is the positive or negative effect those adult practices and actions have on students.*

classroom culture and climate are the antecedents to most student behaviors, both bad and good.

Obviously, these are not "normal times." Even with a positive, healthy classroom culture and climate, the antecedents to many classroom behaviors will have been in play long before students arrived on campus. Add to this the effect of stress on behavior. Continuous and/or high levels of stress can cause intense anger and irrational outbursts. It can cause social withdrawal, sleep issues, chronic fatigue, and physical pain. It can drive tobacco, alcohol, and drug use. The point is that the behaviors and responses that students can or cannot control will be different this year. Which means, as teachers, how we respond and react should also be different.

If a student overreacts or responds inappropriately in class, do NOT take it personally. No matter what the student says or does, they are not actually saying or doing it to you. You just happen to be the random body in front of them at that time. Stay calm. If possible, remove the student from the audience or the audience from the student. Do NOT try to process or reason with the student at this time. At best, this will have no effect. At worst, it will exacerbate the situation. Instead, provide the student with some space and cool down time. Ask the student to look up, to actually focus on the ceiling. This simple exercise can quickly calm a person. Provide the student with some water to drink. Then wait. Let the hormones and chemicals flooding through the student's blood stream dilute. Let the fight or flight response dissipate. Let the overwhelming stress diminish. The student may fall asleep. That is okay, just wait.

When the student has calmed down and can process, talk about their behavior and actions. Talk about what they could have done instead. Talk about what they should do in the future. Have the student practice the appropriate behavior and response. The student should apologize to the aggrieved party or parties, and that apology may need to be written down and practiced. It is possible that reasonable and proportional restitution may be in order. After an incident of student misbehavior, the overriding goals are to reduce the chance of the misbehavior being repeated, repair any damaged relationships, and reduce the amount of time that student is out of the classroom. Class time and exposure to quality instruction will be limited this school year, and there is no guarantee that a school will remain open for the entire year. Further reducing that class time by removing a student from the classroom for an extended period has the potential of causing lasting harm to that student.

A vibrant, healthy classroom community creates a sense of belonging and safety for both student and teacher. Purposefully build this. As a class, process together, work together, celebrate together, and overcome together. Replace the prevailing, singular, and excluding concepts of *I, you, and them* with **us and we**. Then start teaching.

What can one teacher do? A lot!

Chapter 7

FACE-TO-FACE INSTRUCTION

The classroom is set up in a hygienic manner. Students are scanned prior to entering the classroom to prevent symptomatic Covid-19 infectees from spreading the virus. The teacher leads the class in regular and on-going preventive health and hygiene practices. The teacher is attentive to student emotional needs and purposefully builds a nurturing classroom community. For any other school year, these would represent significant overall accomplishments. This year, this represents the to-do list for the first three days students are back on campus.

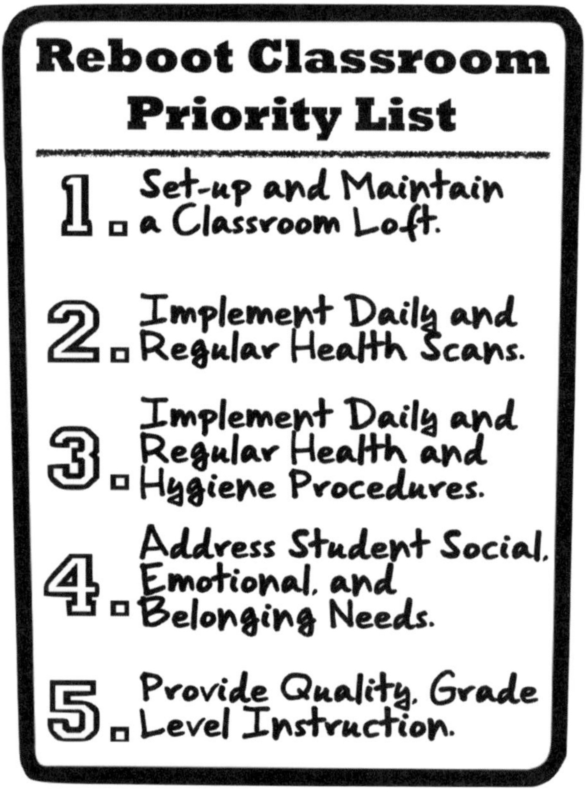

We engage in and fulfill the first four items of the priority list illustrated in figure 7.1 so at some point, hopefully sooner rather than later, we can resume doing what we love most about our job: teaching our content to our students, face-to-face. As is the case with every other aspect of operating a school and managing a classroom, face-to-face instruction will be different this year. To be effective, teacher practice will need to evolve. This will involve letting go of some opinions and instructional

Reboot Classroom Priority List

1. ☐ Set-up and Maintain a Classroom Loft.

2. ☐ Implement Daily and Regular Health Scans.

3. ☐ Implement Daily and Regular Health and Hygiene Procedures.

4. ☐ Address Student Social, Emotional, and Belonging Needs.

5. ☐ Provide Quality, Grade Level Instruction.

Figure 7.1

routines and leaning into new understandings and new instructional habits. The good news is that veteran teachers will be familiar with these new understandings and practices, so their implementation curve can be accelerated. For new teachers, this will be easy… That is our story and we are sticking to it.

We cannot emphasize enough that when students return to the classroom, health and hygiene will take precedence over instruction. Meeting student social and emotional needs will take precedence over instruction. As Maslow's Hierarchy of Needs so effectively illustrates, until our students' needs for safety and belonging are adequately addressed, teaching will be frustrating, and learning will remain difficult.

Students returning to the classroom will be further behind than what has typically been experienced. This will not be due to the "lost" spring semester. In actuality, what was "lost" during the spring semester was primarily content review; teacher, campus, district, state, and national testing; and non-academic activities. The vast majority of new content instruction was completed prior to the school closures that occurred in the last half of March 2020.[4]

Instead, the primary reason why more students will have gaps in understanding, and why those gaps will be both deeper and more widespread, is regression. When students return it will have been anywhere from five to seven months (possibly longer for some students) since they last sat in a classroom. Add to this the facts that time devoted to instruction during the day will be reduced and any given day could be the last day of face-to-face instruction for an undetermined amount of time. As previously stated, in order to be effective, instructional practices must evolve.

Let us start with preparation. Never has a common scope and sequence been as critical as it will be when instruction resumes. Content extensions, enrichment, and deviations were instructional luxuries when there was seemingly unlimited time to teach a subject. Instructional time is no longer unlimited. As such, the scope and sequence should be reviewed for the purpose of **identifying the most critical content concepts** that should be taught. These identified critical concepts drive new content instruction this year. In doing this, educators are reminded to let go of the trope that everything in the scope and sequence is critical. To paraphrase George Or-

---

[4] For a more in-depth explanation of the "lost" semester, see *The Reboot: School Operations in an Unpredictable World* (2020), Sean Cain and Mike Laird.

well, *if all concepts in the scope and sequence are critical, then some concepts are more critical than others.*[5] Concepts that are of lesser importance (they exist) should be moved towards the end of the year and taught if time allows. By doing this, if the school year is truncated, students will have at least been taught what is most critical for overall content understanding. This will address what new content should be taught going forward. However, the question remains, *What should be done to address regression?*

What should **NOT** be done is to take multiple weeks reteaching last year's spring content. Students will already be dealing with greater than normal regression gaps. By not beginning by teaching new content in an expedited manner, then every day spent teaching last year's content increases the distance students are behind in understanding current grade level content. This self-inflicted current year exposure and understanding gap is equal to the length of time of the prior year review period.

Instead, a teacher's best strategy for addressing student regression while teaching forward is to embed a strategic warm-up in every lesson. With a strategic warm-up, the teacher identifies the prior concept that students most need to be familiar with if they are to successfully master the new concept that will be taught. The teacher then reviews or reteaches the identified prior concept as a warm-up activity.[6] This practice of daily, quick, and strategic content spiraling is the most efficient strategy to back fill regression gaps for the greatest number of students, while allowing the teacher to make acceptable progress teaching new content. Note the term *acceptable* progress. Acceptable does not mean anticipated or expected. Anticipated and expected progress is achieved when all of the content delineated in the common scope and sequence is covered by the teacher and mastered by the student. This is difficult to achieve in the best of instructional conditions. This year will not be the best of instructional conditions. Stay alive, keep students healthy, contribute in the efforts to keep the school open, then backfill understanding gaps on the fly while teaching forward. For the teacher who is able to do all of these things this year, they are making acceptable progress.

Once the teacher has identified the new content concept to teach, what

---

[5] George Orwell, *Animal Farm* (1945)

[6] In a typical school year, a warm-up activity should generally take no longer than five minutes. When school resumes this year, anticipate that some (but not all) strategic warm-up activities may take up to ten minutes to complete.

prior content to review, and has completed the daily strategic warm-up, then the face-to-face delivery of new content instruction can begin. Instructional time will be limited this year, both by design and by chance. Due to this, effective teachers will use a wider array of high yield instructional strategies and also use those strategies with greater frequency. Of the high yield instructional strategies available for teachers to consider, it is our recommendation that teachers focus on embedding the highest yield of high yield instructional strategies—those that have the greatest positive impact on student performance. *The Fundamental 5: The Formula for Quality Instruction* lays out five exceedingly high yield instructional practices that, when used consistently and as a cohesive unit, increase student success.[7] The five practices—frame the lesson; work in the power zone; recognize and reinforce; frequent, small group, purposeful talk; and critical writing—are a good place to start when deciding which practices to emphasize when students return to the classroom. The following is a brief overview of each of these fundamental high yield practices.

Framing the Lesson is a practice that should remain unchanged by any Covid-19 accommodations that teachers can expect to make. Every day teachers should frame their lessons correctly, for the purpose of improving student success and retention. A lesson frame is comprised of two statements, an objective and a close. The objective is simply a brief explanation of what will be learned during the day's lesson. Note: The objective is not the lesson activity. The objective is the topic the lesson activity should teach.

The close is a brief statement that tells the student how they will articulate the lesson's key understanding or connection made at the end of the lesson. In other words, the close lets students know how they will demonstrate that they actually learned what they were supposed to learn. Note: The close is not the lesson activity. The close is the proof of connection or understanding that the student gained from engaging in the lesson activity. The lesson frame is posted on the board. When the class begins, the teacher reads the lesson frame and starts the lesson. Then, and this is the most critical component, with two to five minutes remaining in the class, the teacher has students cease the lesson activity and engage in the close.[8]

---

[7] *The Fundamental 5: The Formula for Quality Instruction (2011)*, Sean Cain and Mike Laird.

[8] The timing of the close may need to be adjusted to accommodate end of class cleaning and sanitizing activities.

It is just that simple, and when done correctly will be the most powerful practice the teacher uses that day.

When the teacher begins the lesson by using a lesson frame, it primes the student to be more receptive to learning and provides the student with some context and purpose. At the end of the class when the teacher closes the lesson correctly, it significantly improves student retention of the material. If at the end of every lesson a student remembers a little more of what was taught that day, the teacher can spend less time reteaching and reviewing just taught content the next day. This allows the teacher to devote more class time to covering new material, which means that students are exposed to more content. When every instructional minute is valuable and any instructional day may be the last, covering more content while maximizing student reception to instruction and retention of concepts is paramount.

Working in the power zone is proximity teaching and monitoring by the teacher. With face masks, face shields, and increased physical distancing, working in the power zone will look and feel different this year, but the concept remains unchanged. Teachers will need to be aware of when they touch a student's desk and work materials. They should consciously attempt to do so less often and wash their hands multiple times every class. Teachers have never been expected to spend the entire class period in the power zone. This is neither realistic nor possible. This year, it can be anticipated that teachers will spend less time working in the power zone. However, teachers should still endeavor to work in the power zone when this can be accomplished in a safe manner. When teachers are in the power zone, student attention and focus increase while off-task behavior decreases. Without realizing they are doing so, teachers working in the power zone make continuous micro-adjustments to their instruction, which leverages the effectiveness of lesson activities and by extension increases overall student success. When teachers spend more time in the power zone, it is often observed that the overall climate of the classroom is enhanced. Our suggestion is that teachers reduce the amount of time they actually spend in the power zone but increase the number of times they are there during class. This means that instead of spending a continuous fifteen or twenty minutes in the power zone lecturing to or generally monitoring the class, the teacher now lectures and monitors from the front of the room (an admittedly less effective practice) and purposefully and expeditiously checks on students at their desk two to four times during the class.

Recognition and reinforcement remains unchanged and is another powerful instructional strategy. It is the personal and specific recognition of student academic success and growth and the personal and specific reinforcement of student effort and persistence when faced with adversity. The better teachers are at providing authentic recognition and reinforcement, the more students try and the longer they stay engaged. Extra effort on the part of the student can be and often is the difference between success and failure. The effective use of recognition and reinforcement has a powerful and positive impact on classroom climate. An increase in authentic recognition and reinforcement strengthens the personal bond between teacher and student and helps build student self-confidence. An increased level of authentic recognition and reinforcement is positively correlated to time spent by the teacher in the power zone. The more time teachers spend in close, now hygienically appropriate, proximity to students while they are working, the more opportunities for the teacher to notice student effort and improvement and point that out to them. Given the increased social and emotional needs of students when they return, this practice will be even more important than in the past.

Frequent, small group, purposeful talk about the learning will look different this year. However, it will remain a powerful instructional strategy that allows students to process information, fill in gaps in understanding, and retain information more effectively and efficiently. Teachers who use this strategy with great success realize that if students are unable to talk about a concept, then they often struggle to truly understand the concept. Frequent, small group, purposeful talk also helps students build and add to their academic vocabulary while providing authentic opportunities to think deeper about content (rigor). As is the case with power zone implementation, there are some considerations that should be taken into account. Students should be spaced further apart and now "**small group**" means "**a single partner**." Students should also have a limited number of talking partners per class, per day. In a self-contained classroom, this may mean that a student has the same talking partner all day long. In a single content class, the student has one talking partner for that class. Talking partners can be switched on a daily or weekly basis.

When this practice (purposeful talk) can be safely implemented, teachers should consider allowing students to confer with a partner when working on formative assignments. When students are allowed to confer with a partner on formative assignments, they often backfill gaps in their understanding more efficiently and master new material at a quicker pace. It is a given that students will have deeper and more widespread deficits in understanding when schools reopen. Allowing students to confer with a partner as they work will position students to support each other, increase student success, increase the instructional pace of the classroom, and reduce the stress faced by teachers when they are the sole source of knowledge in the classroom. **Before teachers have students engage in purposeful talk and/or allow them to confer on a regular basis, face mask wearing, frequent handwashing, and sanitizing desks and materials must become regularly occurring, in-class rituals.**

Critical writing represents the most powerful instructional strategy available to teachers. The correct implementation of this practice will essentially remain unchanged when school resumes. This powerful practice is observed in typical classrooms less than 5% of the time. This does not mean that students never write. It means that teachers have students write critically on an infrequent basis. Many teachers do not realize that there is a distinction between critical writing and pencil on paper activities. Critical writing is writing for the specific purpose of increasing cognition and connections. When students write critically, instructional rigor is enhanced, and retention is increased more efficiently than with any other instructional practice. Students who write critically more often will enjoy more academic success than their peers. Due to these facts, when students return to the classroom, every teacher should embed significantly more critical writing activities in their lessons. There should be at least one critical writing activity in every lesson, every day. Critical writing does not have length, format, grammar, punctuation, or spelling requirements. What is required for critical writing is proof of thinking and/or connection of ideas. Critical writing can be informal, quick, and even messy, or it can be formal, long, and polished. The teachers that embed the most critical writing in their classroom rely heavily on the quick, messy, and informal version—the critical quick write. A critical quick write can be used as a warm-up activity or to replace lesser lesson tasks, and it works exceptionally well as the lesson closure. Any lesson without a critical writing component is a lesson that is less effective than it could be.

When possible, especially in classrooms without exterior windows or classrooms that have windows that do not open, instruction and class activities should occur outside. Outside instruction lends itself to improved social distancing, provides unlimited volumes of fresh air, and enjoys enhanced air circulation. As such, outside instruction represents another concrete example of rolling the die less. We understand that every class cannot be taught outside every day. We suggest that teachers

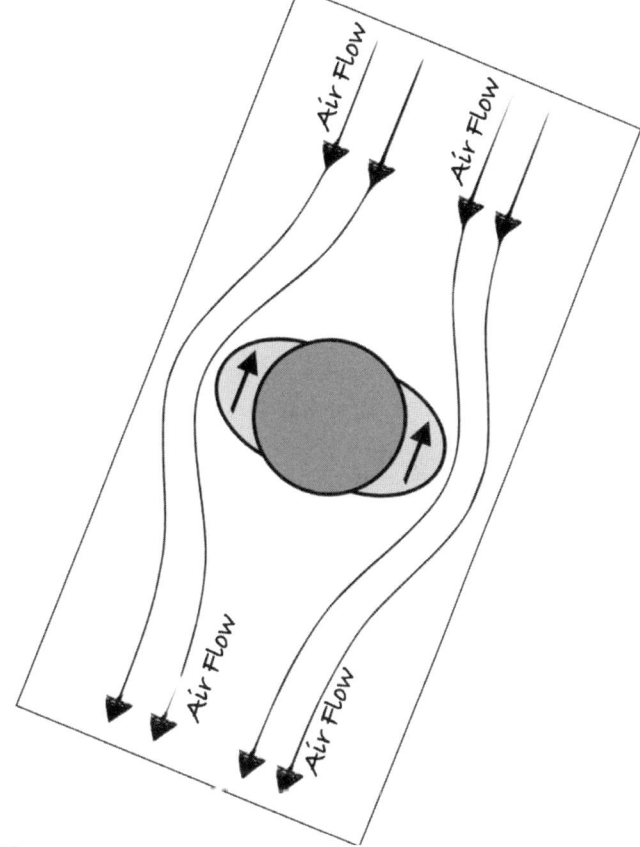

Figure 7.2

be strategic in their use of outdoor instruction. Do not plan on spending the entire class period outside, spend some time outside. Take students outside for the lecture portion of the lesson, or the independent reading segment, or the independent practice time. Students can sit against a campus exterior wall as they listen, read, talk, and/or work. Outside instructional space does not need to be fancy or exceedingly comfortable. It is the space for distancing, volumes of fresh air, air circulation, and natural light that makes this practice desirable.

If a lesson requires students to confer for an extended period of time or engage in a group discussion, talking to each other outside would be more healthy and hygienic than doing so inside. We also recommend adding the additional step of having students walk as they talk. The science behind this recommendation is basic aerodynamics. As a large, heavy body (a person) pushes through the air, the much smaller, lighter virus particles do not land on the person. Instead they flow around the person. The effect is illustrated in figure 7.2. As such, adopting this new rule of thumb would be useful: ***If we are going to talk, we need to walk.***

This year, every day of face-to-face instruction should be considered a gift. Treat it as such. Implementing classroom health and hygiene practices on a daily basis allows us to extend the length of time we can enjoy this gift. Being attentive to student emotional needs will amplify the resonance of this gift. Finally, embedding more high yield practices in our delivery will maximize the positive impact of this gift. We implore teachers: do not take face-to-face instruction for granted.

Chapter 8

REMOTE INSTRUCTION

Many schools will reopen by providing only remote instruction. Every school must plan on having to convert to remote instruction at any time during the school year. Remote instruction, for the foreseeable future, is a fact of life for every school and every teacher. As such, a quick examination of the topic is warranted. First, no matter a teacher's preference or comfort level, remote instruction is less effective than face-to-face instruction. This is not an indictment of the practice, just a statement of fact. Much like the fact that a t-shirt provides less protection against the cold than a jacket. Because remote instruction is less effective than face-to-face instruction, teachers must anticipate that fewer students will master the concepts being taught, and those that do master the concepts will take longer to do so. However, remote instruction is not a hopeless cause, especially when there are no other scalable options available. What we must do is endeavor to maximize the effectiveness of this less effective mode of instruction.

As addressed in Chapter 7, this year it is recommend that teachers identify the most critical concepts in their scope and sequence and focus on teaching those concepts first. When determining what concepts to teach remotely, teachers should review their list of critical content concepts, and identify the most critical concepts on the list. These newly identified uber-critical concepts should be the focus of remote instruction.

Teachers should teach their remote lessons live, while also recording themselves if possible. The only purpose for recording the lesson is to serve as an additional resource for students. With the lesson recorded and available, students can either watch the lesson when they have access to a screen and bandwidth or rewatch the lesson, focusing on areas of confusion and misunderstanding.

When operating in a remote instructional environment, teachers should be available to students at different times throughout the day. Without question, teachers should be available during scheduled live instruction time. In addition to this time, there should also be regularly scheduled times throughout the week when the student can contact the teacher for additional support. Envision something along the lines of posted office hours. At least one of these times should be in the evening, to accommodate students in households where they are unable to have unfettered access to screens and bandwidth.

When designing lessons to deliver remotely, the teacher should "chunk" content. These "chunks" of delivered content should last between three and ten minutes. The maximum length of time of a chunk is determined by the age and maturity of the students being taught. Figure 8.1 provides working guidelines for chunk length by grade level.

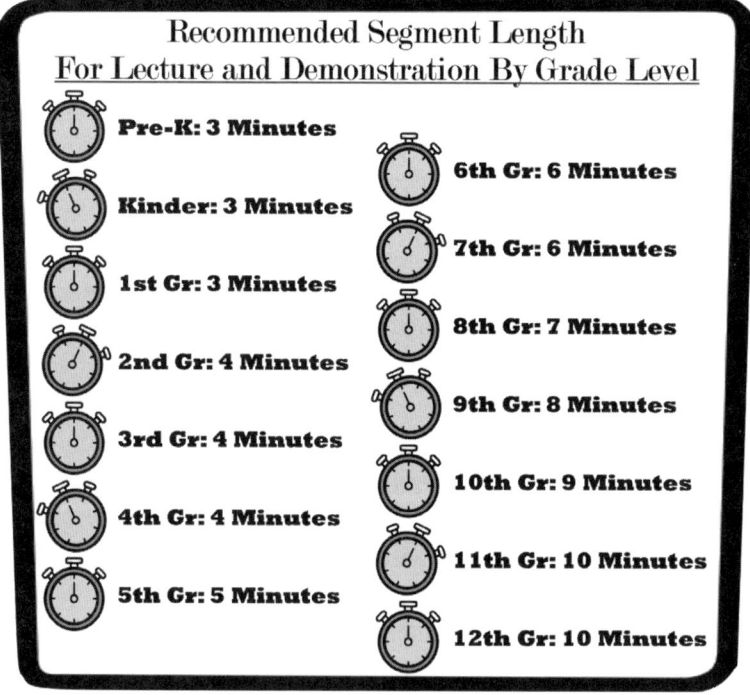

Figure 8.1

When chunking a lesson, after the teacher completes the explanation or demonstration of a major instructional concept or reaches the maximum recommended segment length (see figure 8.1), whichever comes first, the teacher stops. At this point the teacher has the students actively engage in the lesson. This student engagement can take any number of forms.

Students can engage in brief, small group conversations or chats. Students can quickly take notes for a brief period. Students could attempt a practice exercise or problem. The teacher could give the students a brief amount of processing time, and then have them type a question or comment in a chat box. When students complete the (often short) engagement activity, the teacher resumes teaching the next chunk of the lesson. The teacher repeats this delivery pattern until the entire lesson has been shared.

When teachers deliver their lesson in chunks, they are teaching to the maximum limit of their students' attention span and then introducing a state change.[9] When the teacher resumes talking or demonstrating after students complete the state change activity, the students are able to refocus and remain attentive during the next lesson chunk. Teachers who do not deliver instruction in this manner will have students who zone out and will often miss important information and relevant details, even as they seemingly "listen" to the lesson. When this occurs often and with multiple students, it is not a student attention issue, it is a lesson delivery issue.

In the course of the remotely delivered instruction, as is the case with face-to-face instruction, the teacher should embed as many Fundamental 5 practices in their delivery and in the lesson as possible.[10] This begins with the teacher using a **Lesson Frame** for every lesson. The teacher should begin the lesson introducing the frame and if possible the lesson frame should be visible in the footer of presentation slides or scrolled across the bottom of the video. In a remote instructional environment, a written close might be easier to implement than a talking close. Students can respond in a chat box, in a Google Doc, upload their response to a shared server, or hold their response in front of their device camera for the teacher to quickly review. The added benefit to the overall lesson when using a written close is that while a talking close enhances retention and cognition, a written close does this to a greater degree.

There is a model for teachers **working in the power zone** in a remote instructional environment. The model is that of the attentive computer lab teacher. The attentive computer lab teacher monitors the screens of all of the students in the class, ensuring that students are on task and are not experiencing excessive difficulty. The teacher engages off task students by

---

[9] State change: A change in physical or mental state.

[10] *The Fundamental 5: The Formula for Quality Instruction* (2011), Sean Cain and Mike Laird.

gently prodding them back to the appropriate task, provides timely support to struggling students, and regularly checks in with other students to gauge progress and provide encouragement. Physical proximity may not be possible in a remote instructional environment, but enhanced teacher attention and just-in-time micro-adjustments to instruction are often easier to implement.

The delivery of **recognition and reinforcement** may look slightly different in a remote instructional environment, but the intent and effect remain the same. The teacher intent is to facilitate engagement, improve motivation, increase effort, and elevate performance. In a remote instructional environment, teachers can use emojis and images to signify and highlight individual student effort, progress, and success. They can also make the practice more widespread and timely than what is often possible in a classroom. We also recommend the teachers take advantage of chat features in on-line environments to personalize communication with students. The key is increasing the amount of personal and specific recognition of performance growth and personal and specific reinforcement of effort that is provided to students. The short version of the research behind this practice is that teachers who do so have students who try harder and longer, which drives improved academic success. In a remote instructional environment, keeping students focused, engaged, and trying is more difficult than in the classroom. To battle this, the teacher should unleash their inner video game. This means that teachers should share gold stars, thumb-ups, likes, sparkles, and improved score announcements as if they are candy and it is Halloween.

Depending on the platform used for remote instruction, **frequent, small group, purposeful talk about the learning** may still be a viable strategy. What is required is a breakout room feature. The teacher creates breakout rooms in the virtual classroom. Two or three students are assigned to each breakout room. When the teacher completes a lesson chunk (as described earlier in this chapter) the teacher provides the students with a pre-planned question, then sends them to their breakout room for a specified amount of time. The time allotted for the breakout discussion is based on the age of the student and the level of concept understanding. Typically, the time range is from thirty seconds (younger students and/or low concept understanding) to three minutes (older students and/or high content understanding). When the allotted time has expired, the students are recalled to the main room. Many platforms do this automatically and/

or allow for the main user to do it on command. Without a breakout room feature, purposeful talk may be difficult to manage as class size increases. When this is the case, purposeful chat (utilizing a chatroom feature) may be the best viable alternative. Figure 8.2, provides some suggested question stems for different parts of a lesson.

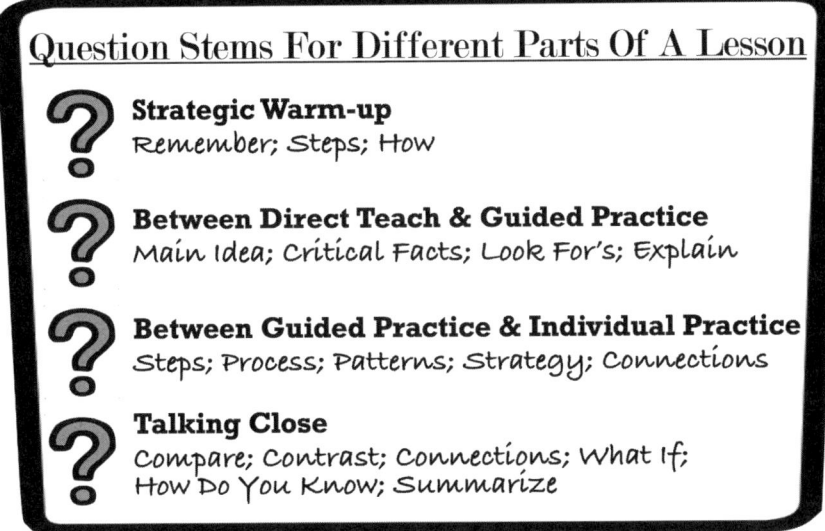

Question Stems For Different Parts Of A Lesson

Strategic Warm-up
Remember; Steps; How

Between Direct Teach & Guided Practice
Main Idea; Critical Facts; Look For's; Explain

Between Guided Practice & Individual Practice
Steps; Process; Patterns; Strategy; Connections

Talking Close
Compare; Contrast; Connections; What If;
How Do You Know; Summarize

Figure 8.2

Not only does **Critical Writing** represent the most powerful high yield instructional strategy, it also easily lends itself to a remote instructional environment. This is especially the case for the teacher who embeds critical quick writes into the lesson. In a remote instructional environment, the teacher should encourage note making by all students. For the teacher chunking lesson delivery, the time between chunks is perfect for notes. Then before the teacher begins the next lesson chunk, students hold their notes in front of their device camera so the teacher can see that notes were written.

The chat feature in most remote instruction platforms is a good vehicle for students to write critically and for the teacher to immediately see the writing. We also suggest that teachers embed the written identification of similarities and differences in every lesson that they can. Variations of this significantly powerful critical writing strategy range from short paragraphs, to a few sentences, to bullet points, to Venn Diagrams, and to T-Charts. In the quicker variations of bullet points, Venn Diagrams, and T-

Charts, students can hold up their completed work in front of their device camera allowing the teacher to quickly check their work. If it is a given that remote instruction is less effective than face-to-face instruction, then it stands to reason that teachers need to use the highest of high yield instructional strategies every time the opportunity presents itself.

On the priority list of schools this year, keeping staff and students healthy and safe is at the top of the list. Further down, but still on the list, is educating students. Remote instruction is a good solution for ensuring health and safety. Unfortunately, for educating most students, it is a marginal solution. Remote instruction is adequate for a small niche of students. It is a Band-Aid for most students. It is ineffective for the remaining student population. Think of remote instruction as emergency rations, calories to be consumed when there is no other option. Remote instruction is not our best instruction. The purpose of remote instruction is to sustain students until they can return to school.

Chapter 9

THE UNSUNG HERO

No matter how much we prepare for this upcoming school year, the only thing we can predict with complete certainty is uncertainty. When schools reboot, things will be different. What we did individually and collectively prior to March 2020 will not be effective without adjustments. Expect this, plan for this. Then do not be surprised or disappointed when we realize that our adjustments need to be adjusted. 2020 has taught us that the best advice, recommendations, and practices from just yesterday can be reversed or discarded due to research being conducted at a full sprint and the high stakes faced during this shared experience. As such, we believe that the best strategy for success in such an environment is to embrace flexible thinking and cultivate an up tempo response cycle. This can be hard, but without realizing it, educators already do this. Good teachers constantly look for new and better ways to improve the outcomes for all of the students in their class. This is real life flexible thinking. Good teachers adjust their practices and intervene when they observe students struggling. This is a real life up tempo response cycle. All that remains is to fully embrace and lean into this. That is the first step in getting though this pandemic.

Step two is to embrace two other characteristics that educators share: intelligence and empathy. Teachers are smart, critical thinkers who truly care about their fellow man and woman. Do not fall for the charlatans and snake oil sellers hawking fake cures and magical thinking. Follow the science and trust the evidence. Reject the false calculus that the chance of dying from Covid-19 is statistically low. While this may be true in the broadest sense, it does not apply in schools. On a campus, the death of just one staff member or student spreads a pall over the school that leaves a chilling effect that lingers for years. That is why until there is a widely available vaccine for Covid-19, the priority for schools is again: **1 – Keep the Adults Alive; 2 – Keep the Students Healthy; 3 – Keep the School Open.**

The best way to meet these priorities is to maintain the operational assumption that everyone is infected with Covid-19, and then implement the practices that would prevent you from contracting the virus. For the educator that follows the suggestions laid out in this book, that is exactly what they will be doing, every class period, every day (see figure 9.1). By doing so, they are not only protecting themselves and their students, they are modeling and teaching the changes in daily behavior that will eventually beat back Covid-19. If we do this right, you the educator will be the unsung hero that jump starts the economy and buys the scientists and doctors the time they need to find a cure.

What can one teacher do? Obviously, a lot!

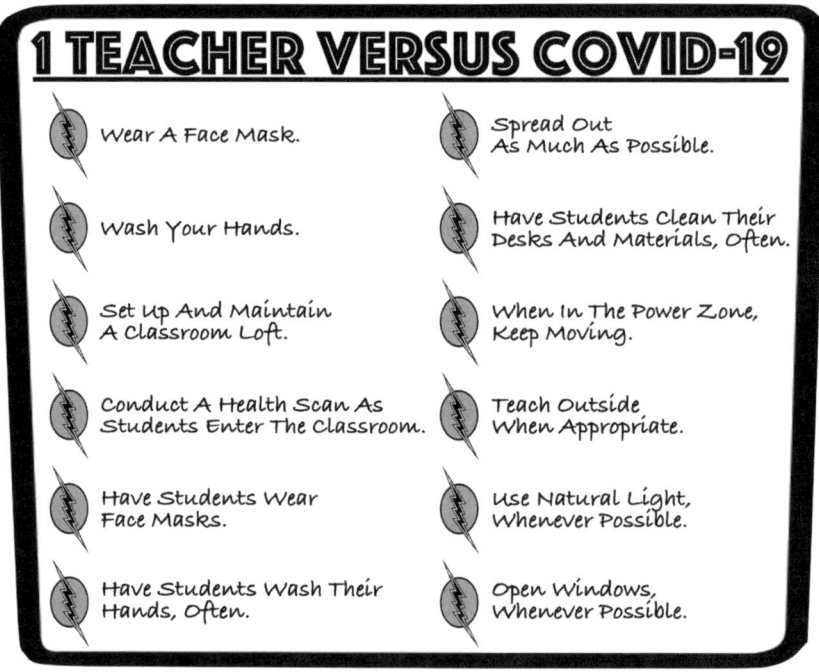

Figure 9.1

Excerpts From *Preparing K-12 School Administrators For A Safe Return to School in Fall 2020*

July 23, 2020 (www.cdc.gov)

Schools are an important part of the infrastructure of communities and play a critical role in supporting the whole child, not just their academic achievement.

This guidance is intended to aid school administrators as they consider how to protect the health, safety, and wellbeing of students, teachers, other school staff, their families, and communities and prepare for educating students this fall.

This guidance is for K-12 school administrators who are preparing for students, teachers, and staff to return to school in fall 2020. School administrators are individuals who oversee the daily operations of K-12 schools, and may include school district superintendents, school principals, and assistant principals.

It is critical that all administrators:

- Engage and encourage everyone in the school and the community to practice preventive behaviors. These are the most important actions that will support schools' safe reopening and will help them stay open.
- Implement multiple SARS-CoV-2 mitigation strategies (e.g., social distancing, cloth face coverings, hand hygiene, and use of cohorting).
- **Communicate**, **educate**, and **reinforce** appropriate hygiene and social distancing practices in ways that are developmentally appropriate for students, teachers, and staff.
- Integrate SARS-CoV-2 mitigation strategies into co-curricular and

extracurricular activities (e.g., limiting or cancelling participation in activities where social distancing is not feasible).

- Maintain healthy environments (e.g., cleaning and disinfecting frequently touched surfaces).
- Make decisions that take into account the level of community transmission.
- Repurpose unused or underutilized school (or community) spaces to increase classroom space and facilitate social distancing, including outside spaces, where feasible;
- Develop a proactive plan for when a student or staff member tests positive for COVID-19.
- Develop a plan with state and local health department to conduct case tracing in the event of a positive case.
- Educate parents and caregivers on the importance of monitoring for and responding to the symptoms of COVID-19 at home.
- Develop ongoing channels of communication with state and local health departments to stay updated on COVID-19 transmission and response in your local area.

The guidance described in this document is based on the best available evidence at this time. This guidance is meant to supplement—not replace—any state, local, territorial, or tribal health and safety laws, rules, and regulations with which schools must comply.

Critical Role of Schools

This guidance is intended, first and foremost, to protect the health, safety and wellbeing of students, teachers, other school staff, their families, and communities.

Schools are an important part of the infrastructure of communities, as they provide safe, supportive learning environments for students, employ teachers and other staff, and enable parents, guardians, and caregivers to work. Schools also provide critical services that help to mitigate health disparities, such as school meal programs, and social, physical, behavioral, and mental health services. School closure disrupts the delivery of these critical services to children and families, and places additional economic and psychological stress on families, which can increase the risk for family conflict and violence. [1], [2]

The unique and critical role that schools play makes them a priority for opening and remaining open, enabling students to receive both academic instruction and support as well as critical services. In order to prioritize opening schools safely and helping them to remain open, communities should consider adopting actions to mitigate community transmission. CDC's Implementation of Mitigation Strategies for Communities with Local COVID-19 Transmission has strategies for community mitigation to reduce or prevent the spread of COVID-19, which in turn will help schools to open and stay open safely. Recognizing the importance of providing safe, in-person learning, communities may also wish to help schools by examining whether additional public or private space, including outdoor spaces, that is currently underutilized might be safely repurposed for school and instructional purposes.

Returning to school in fall 2020 poses new challenges for schools, including implementing mitigation measures (e.g., social distancing, cleaning and disinfection, hand hygiene, use of cloth face coverings), addressing social, emotional, and mental health needs of students, addressing potential learning loss, and preparing for the probability of COVID-19 cases within the broader school community. This guidance provides information about:

- what is currently known about COVID-19 among school-aged children;
- the importance of going back to school safely;
- what is currently known about SARS-CoV-2 (the virus that causes COVID-19) transmission in schools and its impact on community transmission; and
- the ways administrators for kindergarten through grade 12 (K-12) schools can plan and prepare for in-person instruction and minimize the impact of potential closures.

What is known about the signs and symptoms, burden, and transmission of SARS-CoV-2 among children?

Signs and Symptoms
Common COVID-19 symptoms among children include fever, headache, sore throat, cough, fatigue, nausea/vomiting, and diarrhea. [3] However, many children and adults infected with the virus that causes COVID-19 are asymptomatic (meaning they have no signs or symptoms of illness).

Impact of COVID-19 on Children

Collecting and sharing data, including how it affects different places and populations, is important for understanding the context and burden of the COVID-19 pandemic. School officials should make decisions about school reopening based on available data including levels of community transmission and their capacity to implement appropriate mitigation measures in schools. Children appear to be at lower risk for contracting COVID-19 compared to adults. While some children have been sick with COVID-19, adults make up nearly 95% of reported COVID-19 cases. [4] Early reports suggest children are less likely to get COVID-19 than adults, and when they do get COVID-19, they generally have a less serious illness. [5] As of July 21, 2020, 6.6% of reported COVID-19 cases and less than 0.1% of COVID-19-related deaths are among children and adolescents less than 18 years of age in the United States.[6]

Early reports suggest the number of COVID-19 cases among children may vary by age and other factors. Adolescents aged 10-17 may be more likely to become infected with SARS-CoV-2 than children younger than age 10, [7], [8] but adolescents do not appear to be at higher risk of developing severe illness. [9] There are currently a higher proportion of COVID-19 cases among Hispanic/Latino children as compared to non-Hispanic white children. Children and adults with certain underlying medical conditions are at increased risk of severe illness from COVID-19. [10] Severe illness means that they may require hospitalization, intensive care, or a ventilator to help them breathe, or may even die. Children with intellectual and developmental disabilities are more likely to have comorbid medical conditions (e.g., diseases of the respiratory system; endocrine, nutritional and metabolic diseases; and diseases of the circulatory system) that may put them at increased risk for severe illness from COVID-19. [11] Although rare, some children have developed multisystem inflammatory syndrome (MIS-C) after exposure to SARS-CoV-2. As of May 20, 2020, the majority of children hospitalized with MIS-C had recovered. [12]

Data on SARS-CoV-2 transmission among children are limited. Evidence from other countries suggests that the majority of children with COVID-19 were infected by a family member. [13] For example, the first pediatric patients in South Korea and Vietnam were most likely from contact with an adult family member. [14], [15] Published reports from contact tracing of students with COVID-19 in schools from France, Australia, and Ireland suggest that students are not as likely to transmit the virus to other students compared to household contacts. [16], [17], [18] However, more research is needed on SARS-CoV-2 transmission between children and household members.

What is known about how schools have reopened and the impact on SARS-CoV-2 transmission?

Internationally, schools have responded to COVID-19 using a variety of approaches. [19], [20] For example, China, Denmark, Norway, Singapore, and Taiwan all required temperature checks at school entry. [21] Most countries have changed the way they operate to reduce class sizes, increase physical distance between students, and keeping students in defined groups to reduce contacts (i.e., cohorting). [22] Furthermore, many countries have staggered attendance, start and stop times, and created alternating shifts to enable social distancing. In some places this means that only certain students have returned to schools, either by grade range or need. For example, Denmark was the first European country to reopen schools. Denmark staggered students' reentry in waves (e.g., one group started school first, followed by another group at a later date), with limited class sizes and using other social distancing measures. [23] Younger students (under age 12) returned first based on their lower health risk and need for more supervision than older students. Class sizes were reduced to allow physical distancing. In Taiwan, students returned to school with mandatory temperature checks and use of face masks. Rather than national school closures, Taiwan relied on local decision-making to determine if classroom or school closures were needed, based on infection rates. [24]

There is mixed evidence about whether returning to school results in increased transmission or outbreaks. For example, Denmark initially reported a slight increase in cases in the community after reopening schools and child care centers for students aged 2-12 years, followed by steady declines in cases among children between ages 1 and 19 years. [25] In contrast, Israel experienced a surge of new cases and outbreaks in schools after reopening and relaxing social distancing measures; it is unclear what caused the increase in cases and what other mitigation measures the schools had implemented.[26] In summer 2020, Texas reported more than 1,300 COVID-19 cases in childcare centers; however, twice as many staff members had been diagnosed as children, suggesting that children may be at lower risk of getting COVID-19 than adults. [27]

It is important to consider community transmission risk as schools reopen. Evidence from schools internationally suggests that school re-openings are safe in communities with low SARS-CoV-2 transmission rates. [28] Computer simulations from Europe have suggested that school re-openings may further increase transmission risk in communities where transmission is already high. [29] More research and evaluation is needed on the implementation of mitigation strategies (e.g., social distancing, cloth face coverings, hand hygiene, and use of cohorting) used in schools to determine which strategies are the most effective. Such research would improve understanding of the impact of mitigation strategies on the risk of SARS-CoV-2 transmission in schools, and ongoing monitoring and surveillance of transmission in schools could help with timely outbreak detection and prevent wider spread.

Why is it Important to Open Schools for In-Person Instruction?

While opening schools – like opening any building or facility—does pose a risk for the spread of COVID-19, there are many reasons why opening schools in the fall of 2020 for in-person instruction is important.

Schools play a critical role in the wellbeing of communities. Schools are a fundamental part of the infrastructure of communities. Schools provide safe and supportive environments, structure, and routines for children, as well as other needed support services to children and families. Schools play a vital role in the economic health of communities by employing teachers and other staff and helping parents, guardians, and caregivers work.

Schools provide critical instruction and academic support that benefit students and communities in both the short- and long-term. The main role and priorities of K-12 educational institutions are to provide age-appropriate instruction and support students' academic development. Reopening schools will provide in-person instruction for students, facilitate increased communication between teachers and students, and provide students with critical academic services, including school-based tutoring, special education, and other specialized learning supports.

Studies show that students have experienced learning loss during the period of school closure and summer months. [30] In-person instruction for students has advantages over virtual learning, particularly when virtual learning was not the planned format for instruction, and schools may not have the resources or capability to transition fully to virtual learning. In-person classroom instruction has the added benefit for many students of interpersonal interaction between the student and the teacher and the student and peers. [31] Teachers are able to more actively participate in student learning, provide feedback as students encounter challenges, and promote active learning among students. [32]

In-person instruction may be particularly beneficial for students with additional learning needs. Children with disabilities may not have access through virtual means to the specialized instruction, related services or additional supports required by their Individualized Education Programs (IEPs) or 504 Plans. [33] Students may also not have access through virtual means to quality English Language Learning (ELL). [34]

When schools are closed to in-person instruction, disparities in educational outcomes could become wider, as some families may not have capacity to fully participate in distance learning (e.g., computer and internet access issues, lack of parent, guardian, or caregiver support because of work schedules) and may rely on school-based services that support their child's academic success. The persistent achievement gaps that already existed prior to COVID-19 closures, such as disparities across income levels and racial and ethnic groups, could worsen and cause long-term effects on children's educational outcomes, health, and the economic wellbeing of families and communities. [35], [35] While concern over higher rates of COVID-19 among certain racial/ethnic groups may amplify consideration of closing a school that educates primarily racial minority students, there should also be consideration that these may also be the schools most heavily relied upon for students to receive other services and support, like nutrition and support services.

Schools play a critical role in supporting the whole child, not just the academic achievement of students.

- **Social and emotional health of students can be enhanced through schools.** Social interaction among children in grades K-12 is important not only for emotional wellbeing, but also for children's language, communication, social, and interpersonal skills. [37] Some students may have experienced social isolation and increased anxiety while not physically being in school due to COVID-19. Resuming in-person instruction can support students' social and emotional wellbeing. [38] Schools can provide a foundation for socialization among children. When children are out of school, they may be separated from their social network and peer-to-peer social support.

Schools can facilitate the social and emotional health of children through curricular lessons that develop students' skills to recognize and manage emotions, set and achieve positive goals, appreciate others' perspectives, establish and maintain positive relationships, and make responsible decisions. [39]

- **Mental health of students can be fostered through school supports and services.** Schools are an important venue for students to receive emotional and psychological support from friends, teachers, and other staff members. Lengthy school building closures can leave some students feeling isolated from important friendships and support from other caring adults. [40] Schools also provide critical psychological, mental and behavioral health (e.g., psychological counselling, mental and behavioral assessment) services to children who may not have access to these services outside of school. School closures have limited the availability of these services. Furthermore, isolation and uncertainty about the COVID-19 pandemic can create feelings of hopelessness and anxiety while removing important sources of social support. Some students may have experienced trauma through the loss of a loved one from COVID-19. Increases in anxiety and depression may occur when students do not have the structure and routine that being in school brings to their daily lives. Finally, having opportunities to be physically active through recess and physical education can help improve students' feelings of anxiety and sadness. These physical activities should be provided regularly to students in a safe and supportive environment that includes physical distancing and strategies to reduce close contact between students.

- **Continuity of other special services is important for student success.** Students who rely on key services, such as school food programs, special education and related services (e.g., speech and social work services, occupational therapy), and after school programs are put at greater risk for poor health and educational outcomes when school buildings are closed and they are unable to access such school health programs and services. [41] During periods of school building closures, students had limited access to many of these critical services, potentially widening educational and health disparities and inequities.

How can K-12 schools prepare for going back to in-person instruction? Expect cases of COVID-19 in communities. International experiences have demonstrated that even when a school carefully coordinates, plans, and prepares, cases may still occur within the community and schools. Expecting and planning for the occurrence of cases of COVID-19 in communities can help everyone be prepared for when a case or multiple cases are identified.

- **Coordinate, plan, and prepare**. Administrators should coordinate with local public health officials to stay informed about the status of COVID-19 transmission in their community. Additionally, planning and preparing are essential steps administrators can take to safely reopen schools:
  ° CDC's Considerations for Schools provides detailed recommendations for schools to plan and prepare to reduce the spread of COVID-19, establish healthy environments and maintain healthy operations. This guidance includes information about implementation of mitigation strategies, such as physical distancing within buses, classrooms and other areas of the school, healthy hygiene habits, cleaning and disinfection, use of cloth face coverings, staggering student schedules, and planning for staff and teacher absences (e.g., back-up staffing plans).
  ° One important strategy that administrators can consider is cohorting (or "pods"), where a group of students (and sometimes teachers) stay together throughout the school day to minimize exposure for students, teachers, and staff across the school environment. At the elementary school level, it may be easier to keep the same class together for most of the school day. In middle and high school settings, cohorting of students and teachers may be more challenging. However, strategies such as creating block schedules or keeping students separated by grade can help to keep smaller groups of students together and limit mixing. Strategies that keep smaller groups of students together can also help limit the impact of COVID-19 cases when they do occur in a school. If a student, teacher, or staff member tests positive for SARS-CoV-2, those in the same cohort/group should also be tested and remain at home until receiving a negative test result or quarantine. This helps prevent a disruption to the rest of the school and community by limiting the exposure. Schools should

have systems in place to support continuity or learning for students who need to stay home for either isolation or quarantine. This includes access to online learning, school meals, and other services. The same holds for students with additional needs, including children with a disability, that makes it difficult to adhere to mitigation strategies.

- **Prepare for potential COVID-19 cases and increased school community transmission.** Schools should be prepared for COVID-19 cases and exposure to occur in their facilities. Collaborating with local health officials will continue to be important once students are back to school, as they can provide regular updates about the status of COVID-19 in the community and help support and maintain the health and wellbeing of students, teachers, and staff. Having a plan in place for maintaining academic instruction and ensuring students have access to special services is also critical.
- **Making decisions about school operations:** Administrators should make decisions in collaboration with local health officials based on a number of factors, including the level of community transmission, whether cases are identified among students, teachers, or staff, what other indicators local public health officials are using to assess the status of COVID-19, and whether student, teacher, and staff cohorts are being implemented within the school.
- **What is the level of community transmission?** There are specific strategies schools can implement based on the level of community transmission reported by local health officials:
  - If there is *no to minimal* community transmission, reinforcing everyday preventive actions, ensuring proper ventilation within school facilities, including buses, and maintaining cleaning and disinfection practices remain important. These actions can help minimize potential exposure. Schools should also monitor absenteeism among teachers, staff, and students to identify trends and determine if absences are due to COVID-19, symptoms that led to quarantine, concerns about being in the school environment and personal health and safety, or positive test results. Anyone who tests positive for COVID-19 should stay home and self-isolate for the timeframe recommended by public health officials. Anyone who has had close

contact with someone who has tested positive or is symptomatic for COVID-19 should be tested and stay home until receiving a negative result, or stay home and monitor for symptoms.

- If there is *minimal to moderate* community transmission, schools should follow the actions listed above, and continue implementing mitigation strategies such as social distancing, use of cloth faced coverings, reinforcing everyday preventive actions, and maintaining cleaning and disinfection. This also can include ensuring that student and staff groupings/cohorts are as static as possible and that mixing groups of students and staff is limited.

- If there is *substantial, controlled* transmission, significant mitigation strategies are necessary. These include following all the actions listed above and also ensuring that student and staff groupings/cohorts are as static as possible with limited mixing of student and staff groups, field trips and large gatherings and events are canceled, and communal spaces (e.g., cafeterias, media centers) are closed.

- If there is *substantial, uncontrolled* transmission, schools should work closely with local health officials to make decisions on whether to maintain school operations. The health, safety, and wellbeing of students, teachers, staff and their families is the most important consideration in determining whether school closure is a necessary step. Communities can support schools staying open by implementing strategies that decrease a community's level of transmission. However, if community transmission levels cannot be decreased, school closure is an important consideration. Plans for virtual learning should be in place in the event of a school closure.

° **Did a student or staff member test positive for SARS-CoV-2?**
If someone within the school community (e.g., student, teacher, staff) tested positive for SARS-CoV-2, assessing the level of risk is important to determine if, when, and for how long part or all of a school should be closed. K-12 administrators can also refer to CDC's Interim Considerations for K-12 for School Administrators for SARS-CoV-2 Testing, which provides additional information about viral diagnostic testing. A single case of COVID-19 in a school would not likely warrant closing the entire school, especially if levels

of community transmission are not high. The levels of community transmission described above and the extent of close contacts of the individual who tested positive for SARS-CoV-2 should all be considered before closing. These variables should also be considered when determining how long a school, or part of the school, stays closed. If the transmission of the virus within a school is higher than that of the community, or if the school is the source of an outbreak, administrators should work collaboratively with local health officials to determine if temporary school closure is necessary. Students, teachers, and staff who test positive or had close contact of the individual who tested positive should be provided with guidance for when it is safe to discontinue self-isolation or end quarantine.

- **What other indicators are local public health officials using to assess the status of COVID-19?** Local health officials can help inform decisions related to school operations by examining public health indicators that are used to determine level of community transmission and disease severity levels. For example, indicators such as healthcare capacity (e.g., staffing, ICU bed occupancy), changes in newly identified COVID-19 cases, and percentage of people testing positive for SARS-CoV-2 infections in the community might be useful to determine whether to maintain or modify school operations. These indicators are set by state, local, tribal, and territorial health and healthcare officials, and should be shared with schools for decision making.

- **Is a cohort approach used within the school?** The level of student and staff mixing within the school should also be considered. If students are kept in cohorts to minimize mixing of students, exposure to an individual with COVID-19 may be limited to one particular cohort and not pose a broad risk to the rest of the school. Cohorts that have been in close contact with someone with COVID-19 can switch to virtual learning and stay home in accordance with CDC's guidelines for quarantine and self-isolation, and the school may remain open.

- **Communicate with families, staff, and other partners.** When preparing to go back to school, regular communication should be used to update students, families, teachers, and staff about academic standards, meal program services, and access to other school-based essential services that students and families rely on. Regular communication with families, staff, and other partners should include:

° Updates about the status of COVID-19 in the school and community

° Notification when there are COVID-19 cases in the school (when communicating about the health status of students, schools should take care to avoid disclosing personally identifiable information and should follow all applicable privacy requirements, including those of the Family Educational Rights and Privacy Act)

° Explanation of what parents, students, teachers, and staff can expect when returning to school; in particular, communicating about:

- the importance of staying home when sick and staying home to monitor symptoms if close contact occurred with a person who tested positive for SARS-CoV-2
- considerations for COVID-19 symptom screenings
- types of social distancing measures being implemented
- when students, teachers, staff and/or visitors will be expected to wear cloth face coverings and whether cloth face coverings will be available from the school.
- everyday healthy hygiene practices that will be implemented upon reopening (e.g., students, teachers, staff staying home when sick, hand hygiene, cleaning frequently touched surfaces)

° actions being taken to prevent SARS-Cov-2 transmission in buses, school buildings and facilities

° actions that families and households can take to help prevent the spread of COVID-19

° actions families can take to manage anxiety about COVID-19

° decisions about operational status, potential use of virtual learning if COVID-19 cases are identified among students, teachers, or staff, and

° guidance on caring for someone who is sick and for parents, guardians, and caregivers who are sick

° guidance on how to reduce stigma. Fear and anxiety about a disease can lead to social stigma, which is negative attitudes and beliefs toward people, places, or things

° Families and students who had to make alternative arrangements with community providers to receive services (e.g., physical or occupational therapy, speech therapy, mental health services) during periods of school closures may need additional support and communication to establish a transition plan upon returning to school. Additionally, some families may have experienced significant hardship that now increases the number of students who need or qualify for some services, such as school meal programs. Schools can take actions to identify, support, and communicate with families who need to initiate new services as schools prepare to open. Administrators can work with community partners to plan for additional school-based services and programs during the transition back to normal schedules in anticipation of an increased need for mental health services.

References

1. Capaldi, D. M., Knoble, N. B., Shortt, J. W., & Kim, H. K. (2012). A systematic review of risk factors for intimate partner violence. Partner abuse, 3(2), 231-280

2. Intimate Partner Violence and Child Abuse Considerations During COVID-19. *Substance Abuse and Mental Health Services Administration* . 2020.

3. Coronavirus Disease 2019 in Children — United States, February 12–April 2, 2020. *Morb Mortal Wkly Rep.* 2020;69:422–426.

4. CDC COVID Data Tracker. Accessed on July 6, 2020.

5. Coronavirus Disease 2019 in Children — United States, February 12–April 2, 2020. *Morb Mortal Wkly Rep.* 2020;69:422–426.

6. CDC COVID Data Tracker. Accessed on July 21, 2020.

7. Coronavirus Disease 2019 in Children — United States, February 12–April 2, 2020. *Morb Mortal Wkly Rep.* 2020;69:422–426.

8. CDC COVID Data Tracker. Accessed on July 6, 2020.

9. Coronavirus Disease 2019 in Children — United States, February 12–April 2, 2020. *Morb Mortal Wkly Rep.* 2020;69:422–426.

10. Coronavirus Disease 2019 in Children — United States, February 12–April 2, 2020. *Morb Mortal Wkly Rep.* 2020;69:422–426.

11. Turk, M. A., Landes, S. D., Formica, M. K., & Goss, K. D. (2020).

Intellectual and developmental disability and COVID-19 case-fatality trends: TriNetX analysis. *Disability and Health Journal,* 100942.

12. Feldstein LR, Rose EB, Horwitz SM, Collins JP, Newhams MM, Son MB, Newburger JW, Kleinman LC, Heidemann SM, Martin AA, Singh AR. Multisystem Inflammatory Syndrome in US Children and Adolescents [published online ahead of print June 29, 2020]. *New Eng J Med.* DOI: 10.1056/NEJMoa2021680

13. Rajmil L. Role of children in the transmission of the COVID-19 pandemic: a rapid scoping review. *BMJ Paediatr Open.* 2020;4:e000722.

14. Park JY, Han MS, Park KU, Kim JY, Choi EH. First pediatric case of Coronavirus Disease 2019 in Korea. *J Korean Med Sci.* 2020;35:e124.

15. Le HT, Nguyen LV, Tran DM, Do HT, Tran HT, Le YT, Phan PH. The first infant case of COVID-19 acquired from a secondary transmission in Vietnam. *Lancet Child Adolesc Health.* 2020;4:405-6.

16. Danis K, Epaulard O, Bénet T, Gaymard A, Campoy S, Botelho-Nevers E, et al. Cluster of Coronavirus Disease 2019 (COVID-19) in the French Alps, 2020. *Clin Infect Dis.*2020; ciaa424,

17. National Centre for Immunisation Research and Surveillance (NCIRS). COVID-19 in schools – the experience in NSW. Sydney, Australia: NCIRS; 2020.

18. Laura H, Geraldine C, Ciara K, David K, Geraldine M. No evidence of secondary transmission of COVID-19 from children attending school in Ireland, 2020. *Euro Surveill.* 2020;25:pii=2000903.

19. Melnick, H., & Darling-Hammond, L. (with Leung, M., Yun, C., Schachner, A., Plasencia, S., & Ondrasek, N.). (2020). *Reopening schools in the context of COVID-19: Health and safety guidelines from other countries* (policy brief). Palo Alto, CA: Learning Policy Institute.

20. Sheikh A, Sheikh A, Sheikh Z, Dhami S. Reopening schools after the COVID-19 lockdown. *J Glob Health.* 2020 Jun;10(1):010376.

21. Melnick, H., & Darling-Hammond, L. (with Leung, M., Yun, C., Schachner, A., Plasencia, S., & Ondrasek, N.). (2020). *Reopening schools in the context of COVID-19: Health and safety guidelines*

from other countries (policy brief). Palo Alto, CA: Learning Policy Institute.

22. Guthrie BL, Tordoff DM, Meisner J, Tolentino L et al., Summary of School Re-Opening Models and Implementation Approaches During the COVID 19 *Pandemic* [Accessed July 13, 2020].

23. Melnick, H., & Darling-Hammond, L. (with Leung, M., Yun, C., Schachner, A., Plasencia, S., & Ondrasek, N.). (2020). *Reopening schools in the context of COVID-19: Health and safety guidelines from other countries* (policy brief). Palo Alto, CA: Learning Policy Institute.

24. Melnick, H., & Darling-Hammond, L. (with Leung, M., Yun, C., Schachner, A., Plasencia, S., & Ondrasek, N.). (2020). *Reopening schools in the context of COVID-19: Health and safety guidelines from other countries* (policy brief). Palo Alto, CA: Learning Policy Institute.

25. Reopening schools in Denmark did not worsen outbreak, data shows. (2020, May 28). Retrieved July 3, 2020.

26. Estrin, D. (2020, June 3). After Reopening Schools, Israel Orders Them To Shut If COVID-19 Cases Are Discovered. Retrieved July 3, 2020.

27. Spells A. and Jones CK. Texas coronavirus cases top 1,300 from child care facilities alone. CNN. Published 2020. Accessed July 8, 2020.

28. School openings across globe suggest ways to keep coronavirus at bay, despite outbreaks. *Science.* Retrieved July 10, 2020.

29. Stage HB, Shingleton J, Ghosh S, Scarabel F, Pellis L, Finnie T. Shut and re-open: the role of schools in the spread of COVID-19 in Europe. arXiv preprint arXiv:2006.14158. Retrieved 2020 Jun 25.

30. Dorn E, Hancock B, Sarakatsannis J, Viruleg E. COVID-19 and student learning in the United States: the hurt could last a lifetime. Retrieved July 4, 2020.

31. Fitzpatrick, B. R., Berends, M., Ferrare, J. J., & Waddington, R. J. (2020). Virtual Illusion: Comparing Student Achievement and Teacher and Classroom Characteristics in Online and Brick-and-Mortar Charter Schools. *Educational Researcher, 49*(3), 161–175.

32. Fitzpatrick, B. R., Berends, M., Ferrare, J. J., & Waddington, R. J. (2020). Virtual Illusion: Comparing Student Achievement and Teacher and Classroom Characteristics in Online and Brick-and-

Mortar Charter Schools. *Educational Researcher,* 49(3), 161–175.

33. Petretto DR, Masala I, Masala C. Special educational needs, distance learning, inclusion and COVID-19. *Education Sciences, 10,* 2020;154. doi:10.3390/educsci10060154

34. Granados A, Parker C, Boney L. How is COVID-19 affecting ESL students?. EducationNC. Published 2020. Accessed July 13, 2020.

35. Dorn E, Hancock B, Sarakatsannis J, Viruleg E. COVID-19 and student learning in the United States: the hurt could last a lifetime. Retrieved July 4, 2020.

36. U.S. Department of Education, Office of Elementary and Secondary Education, Consolidated State Performance Report, 2017–18. See *Digest of Education Statistics 2019.*

37. Fitzpatrick, B. R., Berends, M., Ferrare, J. J., & Waddington, R. J. (2020). Virtual Illusion: Comparing Student Achievement and Teacher and Classroom Characteristics in Online and Brick-and-Mortar Charter Schools. *Educational Researcher,* 49(3), 161–175.

38. Fitzpatrick, B. R., Berends, M., Ferrare, J. J., & Waddington, R. J. (2020). Virtual Illusion: Comparing Student Achievement and Teacher and Classroom Characteristics in Online and Brick-and-Mortar Charter Schools. *Educational Researcher,* 49(3), 161–175.

39. Collaborative for Academic, Social, and Emotional Learning (CASEL). What is SEL? Website. Accessed July 4, 2020.

40. Loades et al. Rapid systematic review: The impact of social isolation and loneliness on the mental health of children and adolescents in the context of COVID-19. *J Am Acad Child Adolesc Psych.* 2020; preprint.

41. Basch C. Healthier students are better learners: high-quality, strategically planned, and effectively coordinated school health programs must be a fundamental mission of schools to help close the achievement gap. *J Sch Health.* 2011;81:650-662.

Excerpts from *FAQ for School Administrators on Reopening Schools*

July 24, 2020 (www.cdc.gov)

What can school staff do to protect themselves and others from getting sick with COVID-19?

School staff can take everyday preventive actions to protect themselves and others from getting sick with COVID-19:

- Washing hands often with soap and water for at least 20 seconds. If soap and water are not readily available, use a hand sanitizer that contains at least 60% alcohol. Cover all surfaces of your hands and rub them together until they feel dry.
- Covering coughs and sneezes with a tissue or inside of elbow, throwing the tissue away, and then washing hands.
- Avoiding touching one's eyes, nose, mouth, and cloth face covering.
- Maintaining distance of at least 6 feet from other adults, and from students when feasible.
- Wearing a cloth face covering especially when other social distancing measures are difficult to maintain.
- Cleaning and disinfecting frequently touched surfaces, including tables, doorknobs, light switches, countertops, handles, desks, phones, keyboards, toilets, faucets, and sinks.
- Staying home when sick, or after being in close contact with a person with COVID-19.
- Limiting use of shared objects (e.g., gym or physical education equipment, art supplies, games) when possible, and cleaning and disinfecting these objects frequently.

What strategies can schools use to help students, teachers and staff be successful in reducing the risk of spreading SARS-CoV-2, the virus that causes COVID-19?

Currently, the most effective way to reduce the spread of SARS-CoV-2, the virus that causes COVID-19, is using multiple mitigation strategies in combination. This may include students, teachers, and staff staying home when sick; appropriately covering coughs and sneezes; wearing cloth face coverings; social distancing; cleaning and disinfecting frequently touched surfaces; and washing hands often with soap and water or using an alcohol-based hand sanitizer with at least 60% alcohol. Some of these strategies may be new for students, teachers, and staff to implement in the school setting. Therefore, increased education, training, and having protocols to ensure these strategies are implemented as intended are necessary to increase the likelihood of reducing the transmission of SARS-CoV-2.

Schools can educate staff and families about when they or their child(ren) should stay home and when they can return to school, while actively encouraging employees and students who are sick or who have recently had close contact with a person with COVID-19 to stay home. Schools can teach and reinforce handwashing practices among all students, teachers, and staff. Schools can also use physical guides, such as tape on floors or sidewalks, one-way routes in hallways, and signs on walls to help students, teachers, and staff remain at least 6 feet apart. Schools can implement flexible sick leave policies and practices that enable staff to stay home when they are sick, have been exposed, or are caring for someone who is sick.

Can physical distance between students in the classroom be less than 6 feet?

In general, the closer, longer, and more frequent the interaction between students, teachers and staff, the higher the risk of respiratory droplets being passed between people. Therefore, CDC recommends keeping a distance of at least 6 feet from other people, in addition to practicing other behaviors that reduce the spread of COVID-19 like wearing cloth face coverings, washing hands often with soap and water, and staying home when sick. Additionally, it is important to ensure ventilation systems operate properly to increase circulation of outdoor air as much as possible.

When maintaining 6 feet of distance is not feasible, try keeping as close to 6 feet apart as possible, recognizing that the closer you are, the more likely it is for respiratory droplets to be passed between people. In situations where maintaining physical distance is difficult, it is especially important to wear cloth face coverings. In areas where it is difficult for individuals to remain at least 6 feet apart (e.g., reception desks), schools can consider additional strategies such as installing physical barriers, such as sneeze guards and partitions. Schools can also consider using outdoor space, weather-permitting, to enable social distancing.

What have other countries done when they reopened school for in-person learning?

1. Internationally, schools have responded to COVID-19 by using a variety of approaches.[1,2] Most countries have changed the way their schools operate. These changes have included reducing class sizes, increasing physical distance between students, and cohorting. Many countries have staggered attendance and their start and dismissal times, or they have created alternating shifts of students to enable social distancing. In some places, this approach has meant that only certain students have returned to in-person learning, either by varying grades attending in-person, or varying attendance by need. For example:

   ° Denmark was the first European country to reopen schools. Denmark staggered students' reentry dates (e.g., one group started school first, followed by another group at a later date). Denmark limited class sizes and used other social distancing measures.[1] Younger students (under age 12) returned first based on their likely lower health risk, need for more supervision, and lower benefit from virtual learning compared to older students. Class sizes were reduced to allow physical distancing. Denmark has seen decreased infections among all age groups since schools reopened.[3]

   ° In comparison to Denmark, Germany reopened for older students with students attending in alternating shifts to ensure a maximum class size of 10.[2]

Could reopening schools lead to increased rates of COVID-19?

Evidence from schools throughout the world suggests that reopening schools may be low risk in communities with low SARS-CoV-2 transmission rates.[4] Computer simulations from Europe have suggested that schools reopening may further increase spread in communities where transmission is already high.[4] As schools reopen, more will be learned about the feasibility and effectiveness of mitigation strategies such as wearing cloth face coverings and keeping people 6 feet apart through social distancing. Regardless of the level of community transmission, vigilance to practicing behaviors that prevent spread among everyone at school and taking other recommended actions to plan, prepare, and respond to COVID-19 will lower the risk of SARS-CoV-2 transmission than it might otherwise would be.

What should schools do if a student or school staff member tests positive for COVID-19?

Schools should have a plan to respond if someone within the school — a student, teacher, or staff member — tests positive for COVID-19. The plan should be communicated to parents, bearing in mind privacy concerns. Assessing the level of risk is important in determining an appropriate response. School administrators can also refer to CDC's Interim Considerations for K-12 School Administrators for SARS-Co-V-2 testing, which describes scenarios when K-12 students or staff may need to have a viral diagnostic test.

In most instances, a single case of COVID-19 in a school would not warrant closing the entire school. Community spread and how much contact the person with COVID-19 had with others, as well as when such contact took place, need to be considered. These variables should also be considered when determining how long a school, or part of the school, stays closed. If the spread of SARS-CoV-2 within a school is higher than in the community, or if the school is the source of an outbreak, administrators should work with local health officials to determine if temporarily closing the school building is necessary. Students, teachers, and staff who test positive or had close contact with anyone who tested positive should be provided with guidance for when it is safe to discontinue self-isolation or end quarantine.

What about students and staff (or their family members) who are at increased risk for severe illness from COVID-19?

Some students and school staff (or their family members) may be at increased risk for severe illness from COVID-19. Schools may offer options for staff at increased risk for severe illness that limit their risk of exposure to SARS-CoV-2 (e.g., telework, modified job responsibilities). Schools may also offer options for students at increased risk that limit their risk of exposure to SARS-CoV-2 (e.g., virtual learning opportunities). Schools should establish policies to protect the privacy of students, teachers, school staff, and families at increased risk for severe illness because of age or certain underlying medical conditions, in accordance with applicable privacy laws (e.g., Family Educational Rights and Privacy Act, Americans with Disabilities Act). Schools may also consider planning for life events and circumstances that can affect students and staff members (e.g., unexpectedly caring for a family member at increased risk for severe illness).

At what point should schools close for in-person learning?
The decision to close schools for in-person learning should be made together by local officials – including school administrators and public health officials — in a manner that is transparent for students, staff, parents, caregivers and guardians, and all community members.

The decision to close schools for in-person learning should take into account a number of factors, such as:
- the importance of in-person education to the social, emotional, and academic growth and well-being of students;
- the level of community transmission;
- whether cases have been identified among students and staff;
- other indicators that local public health officials are using to assess the status of COVID-19 in their area; and
- whether student and staff cohorts have been implemented within the school, which would allow for the quarantining of affected cohorts rather than full school closure.

References

1. Melnick, H., & Darling-Hammond, L. (with Leung, M., Yun, C., Schachner, A., Plasencia, S., & Ondrasek, N.). (2020). *Reopening schools in the context of COVID-19: Health and safety guidelines from other countries* (policy brief). Palo Alto, CA: Learning Policy Institute.

2. Guthrie BL. Tordoff DM, Meisner J, Tolentino L et al., Summary of School Re-Opening Models and Implementation Approaches During the COVID 19 Pandemic. [18 Pages, 2 MB] Global Health

at University of Washington. Published July 6, 2020. Accessed July 23, 2020.

3. Reopening schools in Denmark did not worsen outbreak, data shows. Reuters. Published May 28, 2020. Accessed July 23, 2020.

4. Stage HB, Shingleton J, Ghosh S, Scarabel F, Pellis L, Finnie T. Shut and re-open: the role of schools in the spread of COVID-19 in Europe. arXiv preprint arXiv:2006.14158. 2020 Jun 25.

ABOUT THE AUTHORS

Sean Cain and Mike Laird are the authors of:
- *The Fundamental 5: The Formula for Quality Instruction*
- *The Classroom Playbook: The Power of a Common Scope and Sequence*
- *The Reboot: School Operations in an Unpredictable World*
- *The Reboot Classroom: Teacher Decisions in the Time of Covid-19*

 Sean Cain spent the formative years of his career working in difficult instructional settings. Recognized for the success of his students and the systems he designed and implemented, he quickly moved up through the instructional leadership ranks. This culminated in his last public education position as State Director of Innovative School Redesign (Texas).

 Currently, Cain serves as the Chief Idea Officer for Lead Your School (LYS), a confederation of successful school leaders dedicated to improving student, campus, and district performance. A passionate speaker, Cain is a sought after national presenter and trains educators in school districts across the country. The co-author of the best-selling book *The Fundamental 5: The Formula for Quality Instruction*, he is known for his ability to make complex problems solvable and transform theory into actionable practice.

 Dr. Mike Laird is a retired assistant superintendent, adjunct professor, and U.S. Army Reserve Major. The co-author of the best-selling book *The Fundamental 5: The Formula for Quality Instruction*, his work continues on campuses across the country supporting teachers and mentoring school leaders. A respected national presenter, Laird combines his teaching, coaching, and school and military leadership experience to prepare today's educator to succeed in the modern high stakes school accountability environment.